Pelvic Pain in Women

Editors

MARY T. MCLENNAN
ANDREW STEELE
FAH CHE LEONG

OBSTETRICS AND GYNECOLOGY CLINICS OF NORTH AMERICA

www.obgyn.theclinics.com

Consulting Editor
WILLIAM F. RAYBURN

September 2014 • Volume 41 • Number 3

ELSEVIER

1600 John F. Kennedy Boulevard • Suite 1800 • Philadelphia, Pennsylvania, 19103-2899

http://www.theclinics.com

OBSTETRICS AND GYNECOLOGY CLINICS OF NORTH AMERICA Volume 41, Number 3
September 2014 ISSN 0889-8545, ISBN-13: 978-0-323-32335-2

Editor: Kerry Holland
Developmental Editor: Stephanie Carter

Obstetrics and Gynecology Clinics (ISSN 0889-8545) is published quarterly by Elsevier Inc., 360 Park Avenue South, New York, NY 10010-1710. Months of issue are March, June, September, and December. Periodicals postage paid at New York, NY, and additional mailing offices. Subscription price per year is $310.00 (US individuals), $545.00 (US institutions), $155.00 (US students), $370.00 (Canadian individuals), $688.00 (Canadian institutions), $225.00 (Canadian students), $450.00 (foreign individuals), $688.00 (foreign institutions), and $225.00 (foreign students). To receive student/resident rate, orders must be accompanied by name of affiliated institution, date of term, and the signature of program/residency coordinator on institution letterhead. Orders will be billed at individual rate until proof of status is received. Foreign air speed delivery is included in all *Clinics* subscription prices. All prices are subject to change without notice. POSTMASTER: Send address changes to *Obstetrics and Gynecology Clinics*, Elsevier Health Sciences Division, Subscription Customer Service, 3251 Riverport Lane, Maryland Heights, MO 63043. **Customer Service: Telephone: 1-800-654-2452 (U.S. and Canada); 314-447-8871 (outside U.S. and Canada). Fax: 314-447-8029. E-mail: journalscustomerservice-usa@elsevier.com (for print support); journalsonlinesupport-usa@elsevier.com (for online support).**

Reprints. For copies of 100 or more of articles in this publication, please contact the Commercial Reprints Department, Elsevier Inc., 360 Park Avenue South, New York, New York 10010-1710. Tel.: 212-633-3874; Fax: 212-633-3820; E-mail: reprints@elsevier.com.

Obstetrics and Gynecology Clinics of North America is also published in Spanish by McGraw-Hill Interamericana Editores S.A., P.O. Box 5-237, 06500, Mexico; in Portuguese by Reichmann and Affonso Editores, Rio de Janeiro, Brazil; and in Greek by Paschalidis Medical Publications, Athens, Greece.

Obstetrics and Gynecology Clinics of North America is covered in MEDLINE/PubMed (Index Medicus), Excerpta Medica, Current Concepts/Clinical Medicine, Science Citation Index, BIOSIS, CINAHL, and ISI/BIOMED.

Contributors

CONSULTING EDITOR

WILLIAM F. RAYBURN, MD, MBA
Distinguished Professor and Emeritus Chair, Obstetrics and Gynecology, Associate Dean, Continuing Medical Education and Professional Development, University of New Mexico School of Medicine, University of New Mexico, Albuquerque, New Mexico

EDITORS

MARY T. McLENNAN, MD
Professor, Division Director of Urogynecology, Residency Program Director, Obstetrics, Gynecology and Women's Health, Saint Louis University School of Medicine, St Louis, Missouri

ANDREW STEELE, MD
Professor, Obstetrics, Gynecology, and Women's Health; Professor, Surgery, Saint Louis University School of Medicine, St Louis, Missouri

FAH CHE LEONG, MS, MD
Professor, Obstetrics, Gynecology, and Women's Health; Professor, Surgery, Saint Louis University School of Medicine, St Louis, Missouri

AUTHORS

SUSAN BARR, MD
Assistant Professor, Division Director of Urogynecology, Department of Obstetrics and Gynecology, University of Arkansas for Medical Sciences, Little Rock, Arkansas

ALEJANDRA CAMACHO-SOTO, MD
Department of Physical Medicine and Rehabilitation, Northwestern University Feinberg School of Medicine/Rehabilitation Institute of Chicago, Chicago, Illinois

DOUGLASS HALE, MD, FACOG, FACS
Clinical Professor and Fellowship Director, Division of Female Pelvic Medicine and Reconstructive Surgery Fellowship, Department of Obstetrics and Gynecology, Indiana University School of Medicine, Indianapolis, Indiana

SUSAN HOFFSTETTER, PhD, WHNP-BC, FAANP
Associate Professor, Department of Obstetrics Gynecology and Women's Health, Saint Louis University School of Medicine, St Louis, Missouri

M. BRIGID HOLLORAN-SCHWARTZ, MD
Professor, Saint Louis University School of Medicine, St Louis, Missouri

WASEEM KHODER, MD
Fellow, Division of Female Pelvic Medicine and Reconstructive Surgery, Department of Obstetrics and Gynecology, Indiana University School of Medicine, Indianapolis, Indiana

FAH CHE LEONG, MS, MD
Professor, Obstetrics, Gynecology, and Women's Health; Professor, Surgery, Saint Louis University School of Medicine, St Louis, Missouri

ELIZABETH MARSICANO, MD
Gastroenterology Fellow, Division of Gastroenterology and Hepatology, Saint Louis University, St Louis, Missouri

CAITLIN McCURDY ROBINSON, PT, DPT
Sullivan Physical Therapy, Austin, Texas

MARY T. McLENNAN, MD
Professor, Division Director of Urogynecology, Residency Program Director, Obstetrics, Gynecology and Women's Health, Saint Louis University School of Medicine, St Louis, Missouri

JILL POWELL, MD
Department of Obstetrics, Gynecology and Women's Health; Department of Pediatrics, Saint Louis University School of Medicine, St Louis, Missouri

CHARLENE M. PRATHER, MD, MPH, AGAF, FACP
Professor of Internal Medicine, Division of Gastroenterology and Hepatology, Saint Louis University, St Louis, Missouri

HEIDI PRATHER, DO
Professor, Chief, Section of Physical Medicine and Rehabilitation, Department of Orthopaedic Surgery, Washington University School of Medicine, St Louis, Missouri

MITUL SHAH, MD
Assistant Professor, Department of Obstetrics Gynecology and Women's Health, Saint Louis University School of Medicine, St Louis, Missouri

THERESA MONACO SPITZNAGLE, PT, DPT, MHS, WCS
Associate Professor, Program in Physical Therapy, Washington University School of Medicine, St Louis, Missouri

ANDREW STEELE, MD
Professor, Obstetrics, Gynecology, and Women's Health; Professor, Surgery, Saint Louis University School of Medicine, St Louis, Missouri

GIAO MICHAEL VUONG, MD
Gastroenterology Fellow, Division of Gastroenterology and Hepatology, Saint Louis University, St Louis, Missouri

PATRICK YEUNG Jr, MD
Assistant Professor; Director, Center for Endometriosis, Division of Minimally Invasive Gynecologic Surgery, Department of Obstetrics, Gynecology and Women's Health, Saint Louis University, St Louis, Missouri

Contents

Foreword xi

William F. Rayburn

Preface xiii

Mary T. McLennan, Andrew Steele, and Fah Che Leong

The Approach to Chronic Pelvic Pain in the Adolescent 343

Jill Powell

Adolescents present to outpatient and acute care settings commonly for evaluation and treatment of chronic pelvic pain (CPP). Primary care providers, gynecologists, pediatric and general surgeons, emergency department providers, and other specialists should be familiar with both gynecologic and nongynecologic causes of CPP so as to avoid delayed diagnoses and potential adverse sequelae. Treatment may include medications, surgery, physical therapy, trigger-point injections, psychological counseling, and complementary/alternative medicine. Additional challenges arise in caring for this patient population because of issues of confidentiality, embarrassment surrounding the history or examination, and combined parent-child decision making.

Surgical Evaluation and Treatment of the Patient with Chronic Pelvic Pain 357

M. Brigid Holloran-Schwartz

Treatment of patients with chronic pelvic pain is assisted by detailed history, physical examination, pain diary, and ultrasonography. The possibility of other contributing systems (eg, gastrointestinal, genitourinary, musculoskeletal) should also be addressed and treatment initiated if present. A diagnostic surgical procedure is helpful in patients for whom medical management or whose severity of pain warrants an urgent diagnosis. Limited evidence exists to support adhesions, endometriosis, ovarian cysts, ovarian remnants, and hernias as being causes of chronic pelvic pain. In select patients, ovarian cystectomy, excision of endometriosis and ovarian remnants, adhesiolysis, hysterectomy, hernia repair, and presacral neurectomy may provide relief.

The Laparoscopic Management of Endometriosis in Patients with Pelvic Pain 371

Patrick Yeung Jr

 Video of ureterolysis accompanies this article

Endometriosis, an underdiagnosed and undertreated condition, affects 1 in 10 women and is associated with pain and infertility. Preoperative evaluation should include testing and management of other causes of pelvic pain. Ultrasonography can aid in surgical planning. Hormonal suppression improves symptoms, but should not be used to diagnose endometriosis, and is not shown to be effective in preventing disease recurrence nor in improving fertility. The goal of surgical management should be optimal

removal or treatment of disease and should include measures for adhesion prevention. Rates of recurrence of endometriosis depend on the surgical completeness of removing the disease.

Interstitial Cystitis: Epidemiology, Pathophysiology, and Clinical Presentation **385**

Mary T. McLennan

Interstitial cystitis, or painful bladder syndrome, can present with lower abdominal pain/discomfort and dyspareunia, and pain in any distribution of lower spinal nerves. Patients with this condition experience some additional symptoms referable to the bladder, such as frequency, urgency, or nocturia. It can occur across all age groups, although the specific additional symptoms can vary in prevalence depending on patient age. It should be considered in patients who have other chronic pain conditions such as fibromyalgia, chronic fatigue, irritable bowel, and vulvodynia. The cause is still largely not understood, although there are several postulated mechanisms.

Diagnosis and Management of Interstitial Cystitis **397**

Susan Barr

Interstitial cystitis is a diagnosis of exclusion. The definition has expanded over the years to encompass painful bladder syndrome. It is disease state that is often delayed in its diagnosis and difficult to manage. Treatment options include oral and intravesical therapies as well as both minor and major surgical options. Also, a patient can improve symptoms by following self-management recommendations that focus on both diet and stress management. Treatment options should be periodically evaluated with validated questionnaires to insure they are improving the patient's symptoms, and a multidisciplinary approach is best to manage the patient.

Myofascial Pelvic Pain **409**

Theresa Monaco Spitznagle and Caitlin McCurdy Robinson

Individuals with pelvic pain commonly present with complaints of pain located anywhere below the umbilicus radiating to the top of their thighs or genital region. The somatovisceral convergence that occurs within the pelvic region exemplifies why examination of not only the organs but also the muscles, connective tissues (fascia), and neurologic input to the region should be performed for women with pelvic pain. The susceptibility of the pelvic floor musculature to the development of myofascial pain has been attributed to unique functional demands of this muscle. Conservative interventions should be considered to address the impairments found on physical examination.

Musculoskeletal Etiologies of Pelvic Pain **433**

Heidi Prather and Alejandra Camacho-Soto

Several musculoskeletal diagnoses are frequently concomitant with pelvic floor pathology and pain. The definition of pelvic pain itself often depends on the medical specialist evaluating the patient. Because there is variability among disorders associated with pelvic pain, patients may seek treatment for extended periods as various treatment options are attempted. Further,

medical expenditures for adults for all conditions in the United States. Although there are many treatments, rigorous testing and well-done randomized studies are lacking. Dietary changes and physical modalities such as physical therapy have often been included in the category of alternative medicine, but their use is now considered mainstream. This article concentrates on other sources of alternative and complementary medicine, such as dietary supplementation and acupuncture.

Index **511**

OBSTETRICS AND GYNECOLOGY CLINICS

Foreword

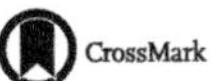

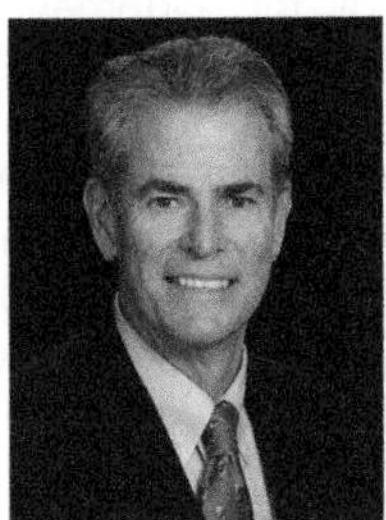

William F. Rayburn, MD, MBA
Consulting Editor

This issue of the *Obstetrics and Gynecology Clinics of North America*, guest edited by Dr. Mary T. McLennan, Dr. Andrew Steele, and Dr. Fah Che Leong, focuses on a condition that is often frustrating for both the patient and her obstetrician-gynecologist. Chronic pelvic pain is defined as pain that occurs below the umbilicus and lasts for at least 6 months. It may be a symptom resulting from one or more different conditions. In many cases, chronic pelvic pain results from abnormal functioning of the nervous system (often called "neuropathic pain").

As described in this issue, a variety of gynecologic, urologic, musculoskeletal, digestive, and body-wide disorders can also lead to chronic pelvic pain. Nongynecologic conditions include irritable bowel syndrome, painful bladder syndrome and interstitial cystitis, diverticulitis, pelvic floor pain, abdominal myofascial pain (trigger points), and fibromyalgia. Gynecologic causes, thought to be present in about 20% of affected women, include endometriosis, pelvic inflammatory disease, pelvic adhesive disease, and vulvodynia.

Because several conditions can cause chronic pelvic pain, it is sometimes difficult to pinpoint the exact cause. Beginning with a thorough history and physical examination of the abdomen and pelvis is essential. The examination should include the lower back, abdomen, hips, and internal pelvis. Laboratory tests, such as a white blood cell count, urinalysis, tests for sexually transmitted infections, and a pregnancy test, may be necessary, depending on the physical findings.

Although therapy targeted specifically to the patient's diagnosis might appear ideal, arriving at a diagnosis may involve costly laboratory and imaging tests and often requires diagnostic cystoscopy, laparoscopy, or colonoscopy. As an example, a pelvic ultrasound examination is usually accurate in detecting pelvic masses, such as ovarian cysts and uterine fibroids. Laparoscopy may be helpful in diagnosing causes of chronic pelvic pain such as endometriosis and chronic pelvic inflammatory disease. If the pelvic anatomy appears normal, the physician can then focus the diagnostic and treatment efforts on nongynecologic causes of pelvic pain.

The authors describe chronic pelvic pain resulting from several gynecologic conditions and the value of treating initially with medications in a sequential manner. For example, if endometriosis is a likely diagnosis, then medical therapy to suppress

Obstet Gynecol Clin N Am 41 (2014) xi–xii
http://dx.doi.org/10.1016/j.ogc.2014.06.004 obgyn.theclinics.com
0889-8545/14/$ – see front matter

endometriosis is given for a trial period. If unsuccessful, then another medication is initiated. Any improvement in symptoms is not an absolute confirmation of a diagnosis, since treatment is often not specific. Hormonal therapy for endometriosis may also improve pelvic congestion syndrome, irritable bowel syndrome, or interstitial cystitis/painful bladder syndrome.

Another medication option is directed at pain relief. Nonsteroidal anti-inflammatory drugs, antidepressants, and anticonvulsive medications are often prescribed. If medications are not effective in treating the pain, a woman may be referred to a medical practice specializing in pain management. Treatment modalities include acupuncture, biofeedback and relaxation therapies, nerve stimulation devices, and injection of tender sites with a local anesthetic (eg, lidocaine, Marcaine). These pain services can also aid women who request narcotics often, which is beyond the purview of most obstetrician-gynecologists.

Either before or after any surgery, pelvic floor physical therapy is often helpful for women with abdominal myofascial pain and pelvic floor pain. This treatment aims to manually release the tightness of muscles in the abdomen, vagina, hips, thighs, and lower back. Other relaxation techniques to relieve musculoskeletal tension include meditation, progressive muscle relaxation, self-hypnosis, or biofeedback. Complementary and alternative therapies are well-handled in this issue.

A small proportion of women with chronic gynecologic pelvic pain is amenable to surgery. Hysterectomy may help, especially when the chronic pain is due to uterine disorders such as adenomyosis or fibroids. Concern exists about pain that persists, particularly in women who are either adolescent or have a history of chronic pelvic inflammatory disease or pelvic floor dysfunction. These concerns are well-described in the issue. A presacral neurectomy to transect some nerves in the pelvis has been shown to be effective for pain resulting from endometriosis, yet this procedure presents surgical risks, so it is not recommended for most women.

This issue serves as an excellent contemporary resource for practitioners caring for women with chronic pelvic pain. I appreciate the efforts of Dr. McLennan, Dr. Steele, and Dr. Leong in gathering a knowledgeable group of authors to cover the variety of gynecologic maladies leading to continued pelvic discomfort. Several sources are described for patients with additional questions. Such patient education pieces answer key questions about the condition as either a general overview or a longer, more sophisticated article. In addition to this issue, the International Pelvic Pain Society and the American College of Obstetricians and Gynecologists provide reliable health information at the professional level.

William F. Rayburn, MD, MBA
Distinguished Professor and Emeritus Chair, Obstetrics and Gynecology
Associate Dean, Continuing Medical Education and Professional Development
University of New Mexico School of Medicine
MSC10 5580, 1 University of New Mexico
Albuquerque, NM 87131-0001, USA

E-mail address:
wrayburn@unm.edu

Preface

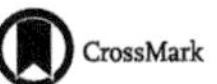

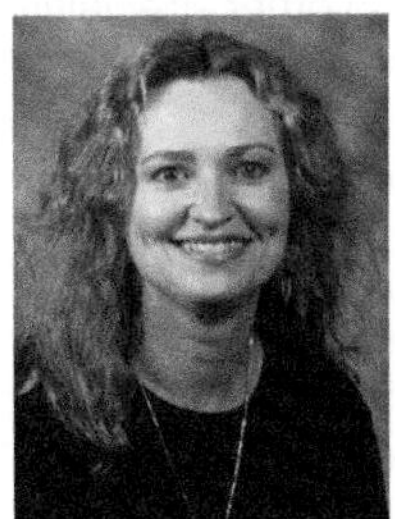

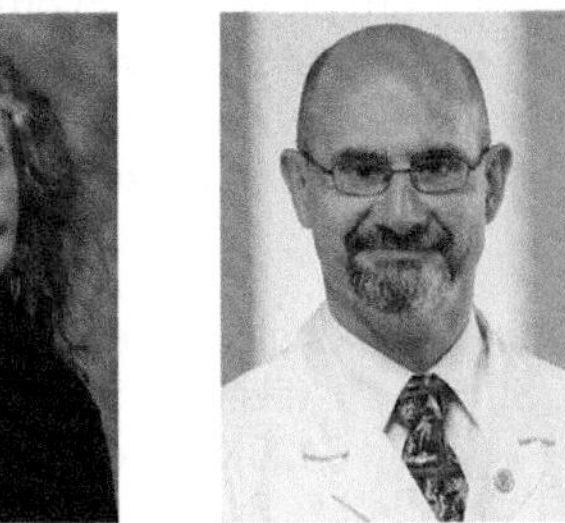

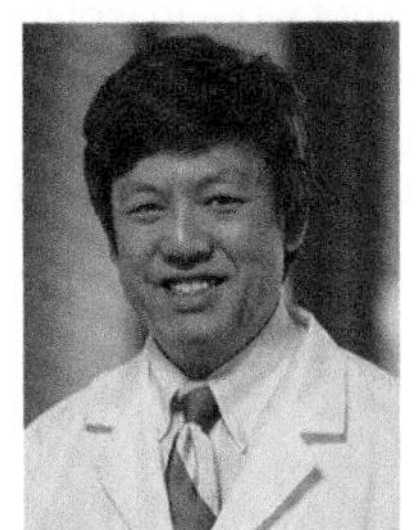

Mary T. McLennan, MD Andrew Steele, MD Fah Che Leong, MS, MD
Editors

Pelvic pain is a very difficult and at times frustrating condition confronting the obstetrician and gynecologist in the office setting. These patients have often seen multiple providers and are often passed between providers with no one really accepting the responsibility of trying to determine the actual cause of the pain. Oftentimes the primary care physician will say it's a gynecologic issue, and the gynecologist will say it's nongynecologic and refer them back to their primary care physician for further evaluation. It is very difficult to estimate the number of patients who suffer from chronic pelvic pain but it is estimated that anywhere between 6% and 26% of patients may have chronic pelvic pain as defined by noncyclical pain lasting for more than 6 months. This can lead to a lower quality of life and lower physical performance. It affects women across all ages and all socioeconomic groups. It is often complex and multifactorial, and unless one has a comprehensive approach to the possible diagnosis, these patients often do not get adequate evaluation.

This issue of *Obstetrics and Gynecology Clinics of North America* attempts to provide an overview of the more common causes of chronic pelvic pain in women. It brings together experts in various fields of gynecology, gastroenterology, physical therapy, and urogynecology in an attempt to discuss the wide variety of common clinical conditions that can manifest as pain. The intent is to enable the physician to consider not only the common gynecologic causes but also the common nongynecologic causes based on certain symptom profiles and targeted clinical examination. Should the physician not feel comfortable in treating the nongynecologic causes, it would enable them to target their referral to a more appropriate physician rather than the patient being referred back to a general primary care physician. It is our hope that it will enable the reader to see the pelvis not as an ovary or a uterus but as a whole system of interacting organs, muscles, and nerves.

Last, there is very little in the Obstetrics and Gynecology literature about the treatment of the pain component with opioid and nonopioid medications. As one of my colleagues frequently states, we can treat the pain but not necessarily alleviate the suffering. The overview of complementary and alternative medications and opioid use will hopefully be useful to the practicing physician as it provides an evidence-based approach to the use of these therapies specifically for chronic pelvic pain.

Obstet Gynecol Clin N Am 41 (2014) xiii–xiv
http://dx.doi.org/10.1016/j.ogc.2014.06.003 obgyn.theclinics.com
0889-8545/14/$ – see front matter

We are grateful to our colleagues from the various specialties who have contributed to this issue of the *Obstetrics and Gynecology Clinics of North America*. All of us need to realize that we do not work in isolation, and there are physicians in other specialties who deal with the same pain issues that we do and that if we have a comprehensive approach and bring together these minds, then hopefully we will be able to alleviate not only the pain but also the suffering for a large number of these patients.

Mary T. McLennan, MD
Obstetrics, Gynecology, and Women's Health
St. Louis University School of Medicine
6420 Clayton Road, Suite 290
St. Louis, MO 63117, USA

Andrew Steele, MD
Obstetrics, Gynecology, and Women's Health
St. Louis University School of Medicine
6420 Clayton Road, Suite 290
St. Louis, MO 63117, USA

Fah Che Leong, MS, MD
Obstetrics Gynecology and Women's Health
St. Louis University School of Medicine
6420 Clayton Road, Suite 290
St. Louis, MO 63117, USA

E-mail addresses:
mclennan@slu.edu (M.T. McLennan)
steeleac@slu.edu (A. Steele)
leongfc@slu.edu (F.C. Leong)

The Approach to Chronic Pelvic Pain in the Adolescent

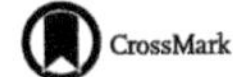

Jill Powell, MD[a,b,*]

KEYWORDS

- Adolescent • Chronic pelvic pain • Recurrent abdominal pain • Gynecologic
- Nongynecologic

KEY POINTS

- A comprehensive history and abdominal, back, and age-appropriate genital/pelvic examination may suggest potential diagnoses or contributing factors, and can be supplemented (but not replaced) with selected imaging and laboratory studies.
- Adolescents and/or parents may want to discuss certain health/social/family history, worries, or mitigating factors with providers privately, and facilitating this opportunity is important.
- Treatment may include medications, surgery, physical therapy, trigger-point injections, psychological counseling, and complementary/alternative medicine interventions.
- Partial or complete outflow tract obstruction is unique to adolescents and causes progressive, often debilitating, pain until diagnosed and treated, and may lead to endometriosis if there is prolonged retrograde menstruation.
- Adolescent endometriosis lesions differ in appearance from those of long-standing adult endometriosis, and are typically vesicular/clear or red/hemorrhagic.
- Establishing realistic evaluation expectations and treatment goals with the adolescent and her family can help minimize doctor-shopping and dissatisfaction, and lead to a therapeutic team approach.

Chronic pelvic pain (CPP) is generally defined as noncyclic pain at or below the umbilicus of at least 3 to 6 months' duration that interferes with daily activities. It is also referred to as recurrent abdominal pain (RAP) in the pediatric literature.[1,2] The differential diagnosis of CPP in adolescents has significant overlap with causes in adults,

---

Disclosure: The author does not report any potential conflicts of interest.

[a] Department of Obstetrics, Gynecology and Women's Health, Saint Louis University School of Medicine, 6420 Clayton Road, Suite 290, St Louis, MO 63117, USA; [b] Department of Pediatrics, Saint Louis University School of Medicine, 6420 Clayton Road, Suite 290, St Louis, MO 63117, USA
* Department of Obstetrics, Gynecology and Women's Health, Saint Louis University School of Medicine, 6420 Clayton Road, Suite 290, St Louis, MO 63117.
E-mail address: powelljk@slu.edu

Obstet Gynecol Clin N Am 41 (2014) 343–355
http://dx.doi.org/10.1016/j.ogc.2014.06.001 obgyn.theclinics.com
0889-8545/14/$ – see front matter

although there are special considerations unique to adolescents such as outflow tract obstruction. It is important for all providers who care for adolescents in primary care, specialty, or emergency settings to be familiar with both gynecologic and nongynecologic causes of CPP so as to optimize patient improvement and minimize medical, surgical, and fertility risks arising from inaccurate or inappropriate diagnosis or treatment modalities (**Box 1**). CPP evaluation in the adolescent poses several additional challenges to providers, including parent-child-provider reluctance to do a gynecologic history or examination and issues with patient-provider confidentiality, as the parent or guardian is generally involved in the visit and medical decision making.

Box 1
Differential diagnosis of adolescent chronic pelvic pain

Gynecologic

- Outflow tract obstruction
- Endometriosis
- Pelvic inflammatory disease
- Ovarian cysts

Nongynecologic

- Genitourinary
  - Interstitial cystitis
  - Urethritis
- Gastrointestinal
  - Abdominal migraine (functional abdominal pain)
  - Chronic constipation/impaction
  - Chronic appendicitis
  - Meckel's diverticulum
  - Hernia
  - Irritable bowel syndrome
  - Inflammatory bowel disease
    - Crohn disease
    - Ulcerative colitis
- Musculoskeletal
  - Abdominal wall muscle strain
  - Abdominal/vaginal myofascial trigger points
  - Nerve entrapment/injury
- Psychosomatic
  - Chronic anxiety/depression
  - Physical abuse or neglect
  - Sexual abuse
  - Secondary gain/fictitious
  - Munchausen syndrome by proxy

GYNECOLOGIC CAUSES

Outflow Tract Obstruction

Complete outflow tract obstruction initially presents with cyclic pelvic pain in a premenarchal, pubertal female. If the diagnosis is delayed, patients develop chronic, persistent pain and may even have urinary frequency, incomplete emptying, urinary retention, constipation, and severe back pain associated with the mass effect of the accompanying hematocolpos and/or hematometra.[3–6] Acute flares of pain at the time of the cyclic, obstructed menses can cause nausea, vomiting, near-syncope, or syncope. It is especially important for providers to consider the possibility of a partial or complete outflow tract obstruction in the differential diagnosis of adolescents with CPP, as delayed diagnosis is common (**Box 2**). This delay can lead to multiple visits to the office or emergency room (ER), prolonged pain and suffering, frequently missed school and activities, and increased risk of future endometriosis if prolonged retrograde menstruation is present.[7]

An imperforate hymen can be diagnosed by gentle visual inspection alone as a bulging, thin, bluish-tinged membrane at the introitus. More proximal obstructions and partial obstruction often can only be diagnosed with imaging. Pelvic ultrasonography is generally preferred as first-line imaging,[8] but for more complex anomalies magnetic resonance imaging (MRI) is useful to fully delineate the anatomy and to determine the appropriate surgical approach and procedure.[9–11] MRI can also be helpful in assessing the kidneys and urinary tract, as many mullerian anomalies are associated with genitourinary tract anomalies, including unilateral renal agenesis and duplicated or ectopic ureters.[12]

Treatment should be undertaken by someone with familiarity and experience with these anomalies. Needle drainage or incision and drainage should be avoided, as quick healing and reobstruction is common and leads to a nonsterile, obstructed genital tract with significant risk of pyocolpos, pyometra, and acute pelvic inflammatory disease (PID).[13] In addition, it is preferable to avoid the use of hormonal menstrual suppression while full evaluation of the anomaly is ongoing, as resorption of obstructed menstrual blood makes anatomic and surgical treatment more difficult. Furthermore, obstruction acts as a natural tissue expander in the vagina, makes septae much thinner and easier to enter and excise, and allows reapproximation of the proximal and distal vagina with less tension on suture lines.[14,15]

Box 2
Differential diagnosis of female genital outflow tract obstruction

Complete Outflow Tract Obstruction

- Imperforate hymen
- Complete transverse vaginal septum
- Vaginal agenesis
- Cervical agenesis

Partial Outflow Tract Obstruction

- Microperforate hymen
- Incomplete transverse vaginal septum
- Uterus didelphys with obstructed hemivagina with associated unilateral renal agenesis
- Noncommunicating uterine horn (uterine anlagen)

Endometriosis

Endometriosis is a common cause of CPP in women, and it is estimated that approximately 60% of adult women with symptomatic endometriosis report having had symptoms that began before age 20 years.[16] It has been found in teens shortly after menarche and even rarely between thelarche and menarche,[17] and was present in 69% of adolescents with pelvic pain refractory to nonsteroidal anti-inflammatory drugs (NSAIDs) or combination oral contraceptives at laparoscopy.[18] It is important that gynecologists and general surgeons be familiar with the appearance of atypical endometriosis lesions commonly found in adolescents (hemorrhagic or red lesions, vesicular lesions),[19] and perform an adequate survey of the pelvis with subsequent biopsy of any abnormal peritoneum if laparoscopy is performed for acute or chronic pain episodes.

Cyclic or continuous oral contraceptives can be helpful either empirically or as postoperative medical management or suppression in adolescent endometriosis,[20] but because of the risk of disrupting bone mineral density formation during its peak time in adolescence, gonadotropin-releasing hormone agonists are not recommended for teens younger than 16.[16] Other hormonal suppression options include high-dose progestins (norethindrone 5 mg 1–3 times daily), progestin intrauterine device (IUD), or depot medroxyprogesterone acetate (DMPA), although the latter now has a black-box warning advising care and counseling if used for greater than 2 years in adolescents, because of interference with bone mineral density.[21] The American College of Obstetricians and Gynecologists now recommends offering long-acting reversible contraception methods (IUDs, subdermal contraceptive capsules) as first-line options to adolescents needing contraception,[22] making the progestin IUDs (Mirena and Skyla; Bayer Healthcare Pharmaceuticals) particularly good options to try in teens who also suffer from dysmenorrhea or CPP[23] that may be due to endometriosis.

Pelvic Inflammatory Disease

As in adults, CPP may result from untreated chronic PID or may be sequelae of acute PID. The Pelvic Inflammatory Disease Evaluation and Clinical Health (PEACH) Study demonstrated that by 84 months following diagnosis and treatment of mild to moderate PID, 40% of both adolescents (age 14–19) and adults (age 20–38) reported pelvic pain of at least 6 months' duration since their diagnosis, regardless of whether they were randomized to inpatient or outpatient PID treatment.[24] A low index of suspicion for PID is warranted, and routine screening should be considered, as adolescents may not be truthful about sexual history, even when asked without a parent present, and are also more susceptible than adult women to PID because of biological (cervical ectopy) and behavioral (sexual concurrency) factors.[25,26]

Ovarian Cysts

Ovarian cysts are common in adolescents, and the challenge for the evaluating provider is to determine whether they are the proximate cause of acute pelvic pain, CPP, or an incidental finding. These cysts are frequently found on imaging done in the outpatient or ER setting for abdominal, pelvic, or back pain, and it is important to review the imaging report and often even the images themselves if the report itself does not contain sufficient detail about the nature, size, or laterality of the ovarian cyst.

A corpus luteum will be found in ovulatory patients about 2 weeks before their impending menses and is typically around 3 cm in size, unilateral, and unilocular, although it may be complex and increased in size if intracystic hemorrhage has occurred. Other simple, hypoechoic cysts commonly found are follicular cysts, functional ovarian cysts, paratubal cysts, peritoneal inclusion cysts, and the classic description of the polycystic ovary syndrome (PCOS) ovary with generously sized ovaries with multiple centimeter/subcentimeter follicular cysts lined up around the periphery of the ovary forming the "string-of-pearls" sign.[27,28] Cysts described as complex, solid, multilocular, or hyperechoic, and/or greater than 6 cm in size, generally require further evaluation or follow-up imaging, as they could represent either benign but progressive processes (dermoid/mature teratoma, endometrioma, benign cystadenoma) or, rarely, borderline or malignant ovarian cysts (germ cell tumors, cystadenocarcinomas, granulosa cell tumors).

Surgery for ovarian cysts in adolescents should be infrequent and should be reserved for persistent, large, complex/solid, or symptomatic cysts, and should be conservative, with the goal of ovarian preservation in most cases, even in rare cases of malignancy.[29–31] In the patient with CPP and PCOS, it is important to educate the patient and parent/caregiver about the pathophysiology of PCOS and its medical, not surgical, management, and to evaluate for other causes of CPP.

NONGYNECOLOGIC CAUSES

Bladder

Interstitial cystitis (IC), also called complex bladder pain syndrome, is characterized by CPP with irritative voiding symptoms, with specific findings noted at cystoscopy. Advanced IC is found regularly in adult women with CPP; therefore it is not unreasonable to suspect that its origins may present in the adolescent or even prepubertal years, although there are limited reported data in the literature about its incidence and prevalence. In a retrospective case series of 26 women aged 13 to 25 years with CPP and urinary frequency who underwent laparoscopy and cystoscopy, 42% had IC, including 4 subjects who also had symptoms suggestive of endometriosis but normal laparoscopy.[32] Importantly this may be underdiagnosed, as it is unclear how long the chronic bladder inflammation in IC pathophysiology must be present to induce the typical glomerulations and Hunner ulcers characteristic of IC at cystoscopy. These findings may not yet be visible in the early stages of the disease.[33]

In adolescents with persistent urinary symptoms (frequency, urgency, dysuria) and a negative urine culture, it is important to evaluate for gonococcal, chlamydial, or *Trichomonas* urethritis by either urine or vaginal/endocervical samples, as these infections will cause a persistent pyuria. In one study of 154 sexually active females aged 14 to 22 years with urinary symptoms who were tested in a hospital-based clinic or ER for both urinary tract infection (UTI) and sexually transmitted infection (STI), 65% of individuals with pyuria had an STI.[34]

Gastrointestinal

There are both organic and functional gastrointestinal conditions that may lead to persistent or recurrent abdominal or pelvic pain in adolescents, including chronic constipation, food intolerances (lactose, gluten), irritable bowel syndrome, inflammatory bowel disease (Crohn disease, ulcerative colitis), and abdominal migraine, more recently referred to as functional abdominal pain. Adolescents are at risk for developing chronic constipation resulting from decreased fiber in their diets, decreased fluid intake during the school day, behavioral conditioning with common avoidance of having a bowel movement at school during the day, and potential diminished rectal distension sensitivity over time.[35] Bowel symptoms with associated weight loss, poor growth, fever, or hematochezia/melena should be evaluated thoroughly, typically including endoscopy and laboratory studies.

One entity that may be underdiagnosed in the evaluation and management of CPP in both adolescents and adults is recurrent or chronic appendicitis. Because of its atypical presentation without rapid progression to an acute abdomen with persistent leukocytosis and fever, it can be overlooked. It may also be inadvertently partially treated with empiric antibiotic therapy intended to treat another potential cause for right lower quadrant pain such as PID or UTI/pyelonephritis.[36–38] Appendectomy at the time of laparoscopy for chronic or recurrent right lower quadrant/pelvic pain does improve or resolve symptoms for individuals with this entity,[39–41] and also eliminates appendicitis from the differential diagnosis. This approach may be helpful to both parents and providers in limiting future ER visits and radiation exposure from repetitive computed tomography scans.

Musculoskeletal

A provider will not make the diagnosis that he or she does not think about, and musculoskeletal causes of CPP commonly fall into this category, as many physicians have little training in evaluating this system. The abdominal wall muscles and fascia, deep abdominal muscles (iliacus, psoas), and deep pelvic muscles (obturator internus, piriformis, levators), sacroiliac joints, and lumbosacral muscles can all contribute to significant pelvic pain. One study evaluated females aged 9 to 20 years presenting to a tertiary care clinic for CPP not explained by gynecologic history, examination, and laboratory or imaging findings, and not responsive to standard treatments for endometriosis. A primary musculoskeletal cause was found in 66% of patients, and secondary musculoskeletal pain was found in 10%.[42] The mean age of those with musculoskeletal pain was 15.27 years and the mean duration of symptoms was 17.97 months (range 1 week to 7 years).

Most musculoskeletal causes of CPP in adolescents are related to chronic microtrauma and biomechanical stresses (poor posture, high heels, leg-length discrepancy, heavy backpacks/handbags, and so forth) rather than acute muscle strain, although certain sports, athletic training, and exercise programs can lead to abdominal wall muscle strain. In addition, myofascial pain can be secondary to CPP from another source. Chronic hypertonicity/spasm in the abdominal or pelvic floor muscles can lead to trigger points: focal hypersensitive, tender, myofascial nodules. Patients may improve with heat, rest, NSAIDs, trigger-point injections (typically with a topical anesthetic with or without corticosteroid), and/or physical therapy.[43,44]

Psychosocial With and Without Psychosomatic Symptoms

CPP can adversely affect an adolescent's school attendance and performance, extracurricular participation, sleep, social life, and interactions with family and friends.[45] These patients may also have signs and symptoms of depression or anxiety, which may be either a cause or effect of the CPP. Tricyclic antidepressants (amitriptyline, nortriptyline) may mediate pain signals and improve sleep, and can be tried at relatively low doses at night. Selective serotonin reuptake inhibitors may also alleviate pain in some individuals and be indicated for coexisting depression or anxiety. Adolescents may also benefit from cognitive and behavioral therapies (biofeedback, guided imagery, and so forth). Psychological counseling can address depression, anxiety, and coping skills, while complementary/alternative medicine interventions, including acupuncture, may improve pain, as demonstrated in 70% of adolescents being treated for refractory pelvic pain at one center.[46,47]

It is also important to consider the possibility of ongoing or prior sexual abuse in an adolescent with CPP, especially in the absence of abnormal laboratory, imaging, or laparoscopic findings. The association between a history of sexual abuse and the development of CPP is well known[48–50] but is often a difficult subject for patients, family members, and providers to broach. It can be helpful to use an intake history questionnaire routinely with any new patients, but especially with the presenting complaint of CPP, to reassure patients and parents that questions about current or prior consensual and nonconsensual sexual activity are routine in the evaluation and do not reflect any judging or stereotyping of the patient on the part of the provider. Intake questionnaires have been shown to be reliable in eliciting a history of sexual abuse,[51] but it is important that the provider follow up on both positive and negative sexual history responses without the parent being present at some point during the visit, as parents may have filled out the form for their child, or the teens may have been concerned about confidentiality if filling out the form themselves.

CLINICAL APPROACH

History

As with adults, adolescents being evaluated for CPP should be encouraged to bring or send pertinent office notes, laboratory results, imaging and endoscopy reports, and any laparoscopic photos and pathology reports for review to determine what is necessary to continue and complete the evaluation without the cost, medical risks, or time involved in unnecessary repeat testing. Building rapport and alleviating anxiety is important and can be optimized by allowing the patient to remain dressed during the history taking, describing the plan for the visit, discussing confidentiality issues, and encouraging the teen to provide input to the history and decision making. Outpatient and ER evaluation of the teen ideally consists of meeting with parent and child together, parent(s) alone, child alone, and then both together again. This approach provides the opportunity for both the patient and parents to discuss concerns, history, and mitigating factors that they may not want to discuss openly. The physician should initiate discussion about sexual history with the adolescent; a recent study reviewing audio recordings of 253 adolescent health maintenance visits demonstrated that in only 65% of the visits was a sexuality issue discussed, and at no visit was a sexuality issue ever brought up by the adolescent.[52,53]

Physical Examination

Examination of the adolescent with CPP should include general evaluation, ideally when the patient is unaware, of ambulation, mobility, and affect. The low back and sacroiliac joints can be palpated to assess for associated primary or secondary back tenderness, which patients often are unaware of or dismiss as unrelated to their abdominal or pelvic pain (**Fig. 1**). Single-digit, superficial examination of the abdominal wall more accurately isolates the abdominal wall as a source of pain before stimulating visceral structures with deeper palpation (**Fig. 2**). If an area of focal tenderness is

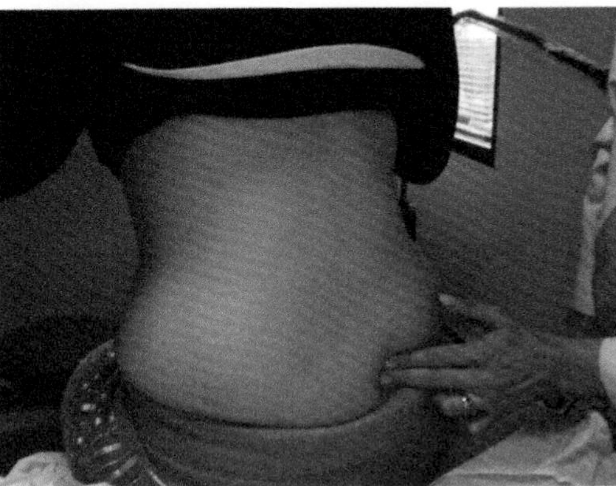

Fig. 1. The low back and sacroiliac joints can be palpated to assess for associated primary or secondary back tenderness.

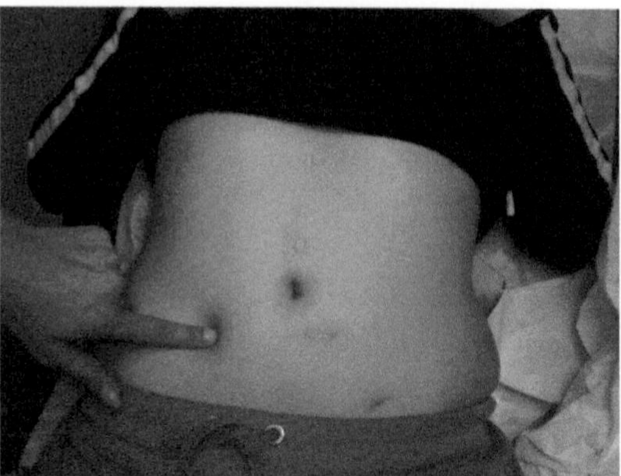

Fig. 2. Single-digit, superficial examination of the abdominal wall.

found, a Carnett test can be performed, consisting of focal palpation of the tender area while the patient lifts the shoulders off the table with the chin tucked to the chest in a "sit-up" maneuver. With a positive Carnett test the pain will worsen with this maneuver, and is more likely to be located in the abdominal wall including the rectus abdominis, obliques, and associated fascia. With a negative Carnett test the pain is improved with this maneuver, indicating that it may more likely be from a visceral source, which is then relatively protected from palpation by the contracted abdominal musculature.[54]

A pelvic examination may or may not be helpful in the assessment, and its feasibility depends on many factors including patient anxiety, expectations about the visit, sexual history, parental expectations, and location and severity of pain. If a pelvic examination is to be performed, it is important to have the assent of the patient and to allow the patient to choose whether to have the parent present or not during the examination. Choice of speculum is important in minimizing discomfort, vaginismus, and anxiety with future examinations (**Fig. 3**). A pediatric speculum will be both narrow and short, but often is not long enough to visualize the cervix in pubertal adolescents. The Huffman speculum is narrow (0.5 × 4 in [1.3 × 10.1 cm]), and is an excellent choice for virginal females or those with a narrow introitus or tight hymen ring. A Pederson speculum (0.88 × 4 in [2.2 × 10.1 cm]) is slightly wider and generally appropriate for

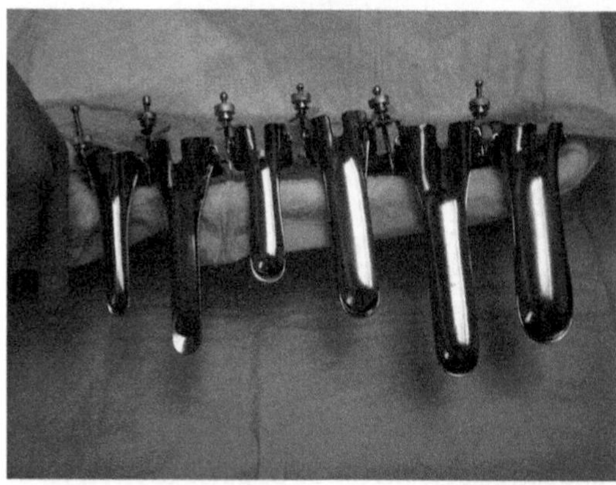

Fig. 3. A wide range of speculum sizes are available for examinations.

nulliparous adolescents who have been sexually active. The Graves speculum (1 × 3 in [2.5 × 7.6 cm]) is generally only tolerated by adolescents with a history of a vaginal delivery.[55] In the patient who cannot or will not tolerate a speculum or digital examination, gentle probing of the vagina with a lubricated cotton swab may be feasible, and can confirm a patent hymen and assess for a vaginal septum. If an STI test is warranted by sexual history or symptomatology (pelvic pain, vaginal discharge, and/or urinary symptoms), it can be performed with either a self-collected or clinician-collected vaginal swab or a first-void urine sample.[56–58] Gonorrhea and *Chlamydia* testing can then be performed using one of several commercially available nucleic acid amplification tests, and *Trichomonas* testing can be performed with either the OSOM

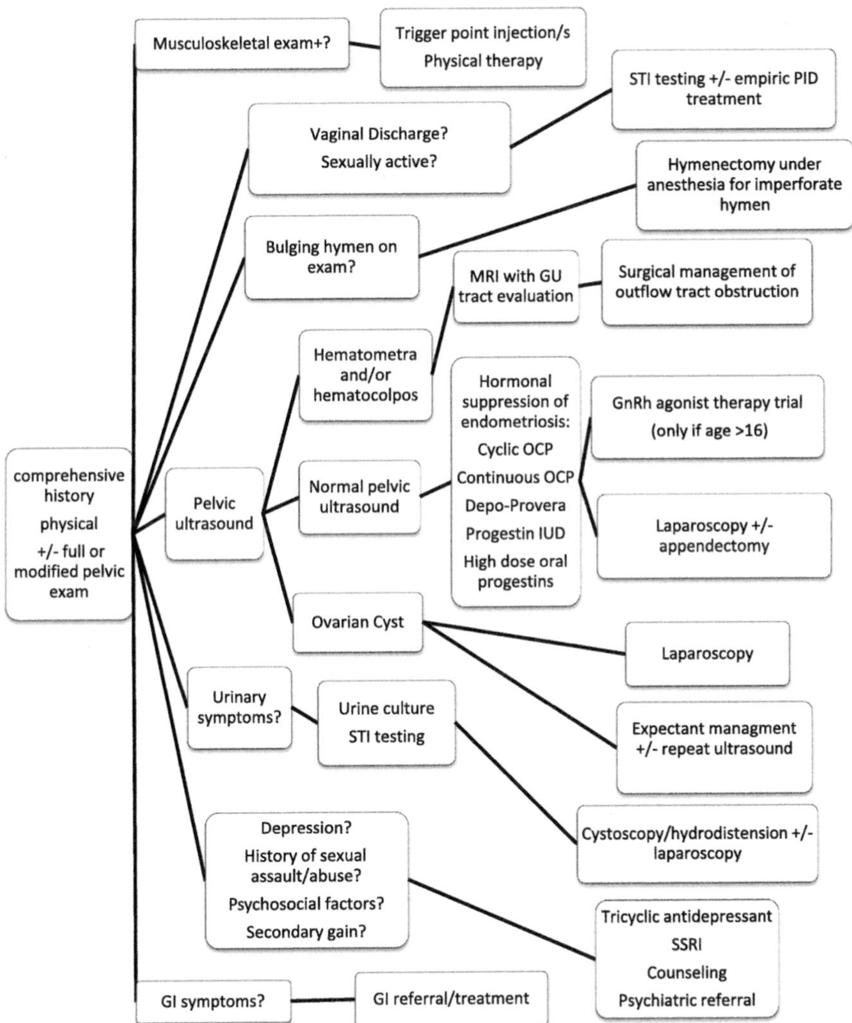

Fig. 4. An example of a care map, sometimes used in treating chronic pelvic pain. GI, gastrointestinal; GU, genitourinary; IUD, intrauterine device; MRI, magnetic resonance imaging; OCP, oral contraceptive pill; PID, pelvic inflammatory disease; SSRI, selective serotonin reuptake inhibitor; STI, sexually transmitted infection.

Trichomonas Rapid Test (Sekisui Diagnostics, Framingham, MA, USA) or the APTIMA *Trichomonas vaginalis* Assay (Hologic Gen-Probe, San Diego, CA, USA).

Following collection of any specimens as indicated, a single digital examination with gentle palpation of the vaginal floor (levator muscles), proximal vaginal floor (piriformis muscles), and lateral vaginal fornices (obturator internus muscles) can be performed to look for increased pelvic floor tone or vaginal trigger points. The urethra and bladder can be palpated for tenderness on the anterior vaginal wall, and the cervix can be gently manipulated to assess for cervical motion tenderness. Finally, the abdominal hand is gently placed to assess the adnexae and uterus with special attention to cervical motion tenderness, ovarian cysts, and pelvic masses.

TREATMENT CONSIDERATIONS

Successful management of CPP in adolescents can be a challenge for providers, families, and patients, and requires an open discussion about the diagnostics, treatment approach, and expectations. Advising teens and parents that the goals are to (1) diagnose any life-threatening, serious abnormality, (2) identify treatable causes, and (3) manage/minimize pain frequency/intensity/disability as much as possible is helpful in setting realistic expectations about treatment goals. Reviewing a list of potential causes of pelvic pain and the diagnostic and treatment steps that may be taken provides a "care map" (**Fig. 4**) for the teen and family, and can build their confidence and trust in the provider and the process. In long-standing, refractory cases, it is especially important to validate the patient's pain and associated frustration and concern about a lack of resolution. Statements such as "this must be very frustrating to you" and "let's work together as a team to get you feeling as good as possible so we can help you get back to school and the activities you enjoy" can be very therapeutic and rapport-building for both patients and parents.

SUMMARY

Evaluating and treating the adolescent with CPP takes time, empathy, and a comprehensive consideration of potential gynecologic and nongynecologic causes. Laboratory and imaging studies are adjuncts to an accurate, comprehensive history and an age- and patient-specific appropriate physical examination. Patients may have multiple, overlapping causes of their pain, and may benefit from the offer of diagnostic modalities or treatments either in a stepwise fashion or, when indicated, concurrently. Discussing diagnostic plans and treatment goals with the adolescent and parent with the aid of a care map can be helpful in building realistic expectations about results and a therapeutic, trusting doctor-patient-parent relationship.

REFERENCES

1. Rappaport L. Recurrent abdominal pain: theories and pragmatics. Pediatrician 1989;16(1–2):78–84.
2. Homme JL, Foster AA. Recurrent severe abdominal pain in the pediatric patient. J Emerg Med 2014;46(5):627–31.
3. Daboiko JC, Gbané-Koné M, Ouattara B. Low-back pain in adolescents: consider haematocolpometra by imperforate hymen in the case of a premenarchal girl. Clin Exp Rheumatol 2011;29(1):146.
4. Buick RG, Chowdhary SK. Backache: a rare diagnosis and unusual complication. Pediatr Surg Int 1999;15(8):586–7.

5. Isenhour JL, Hanley ML, Marx JA. Hematocolpometra manifesting as constipation in the young female. Acad Emerg Med 1999;6(7):752–3.
6. Nisanian AC. Hematocolpometra presenting as urinary retention. A case report. J Reprod Med 1993;38(1):57–60.
7. Dovey S, Sanfilippo J. Endometriosis and the adolescent. Clin Obstet Gynecol 2010;53(2):420–8.
8. Cicchiello LA, Hamper UM, Scoutt LM. Ultrasound evaluation of gynecologic causes of pelvic pain. Obstet Gynecol Clin North Am 2011;38(1):85–114, viii.
9. Kumar S, Satija B, Wadhwa L. Complex mullerian duct anomaly in a young female with primary amenorrhoea, infertility, and chronic pelvic pain. J Hum Reprod Sci 2012;5(3):295–7.
10. Mueller GC, Hussain HK, Smith YR, et al. Müllerian duct anomalies: comparison of MRI diagnosis and clinical diagnosis. AJR Am J Roentgenol 2007;189(6): 1294–302.
11. Olpin JD, Heilbrun M. Imaging of Müllerian duct anomalies. Clin Obstet Gynecol 2009;52(1):40–56.
12. Zurawin RK, Dietrich JE, Heard MJ, et al. Didelphic uterus and obstructed hemivagina with renal agenesis: case report and review of the literature. J Pediatr Adolesc Gynecol 2004;17(2):137–41.
13. Lok IH, Yip SK. Iatrogenic pyocolpos in a young girl with imperforate hymen. Aust N Z J Obstet Gynaecol 2001;41(1):104–5.
14. Quint EH. Severe dysmenorrhea due to obstructive anomaly. J Pediatr Adolesc Gynecol 2002;15(3):175–7.
15. Beyth Y, Klein Z, Weinstein S, et al. Thick transverse vaginal septum: expectant management followed by surgery. J Pediatr Adolesc Gynecol 2004;17(6):379–81.
16. American College of Obstetricians and Gynecologists. ACOG Committee Opinion. Number 310, April 2005. Endometriosis in adolescents. Obstet Gynecol 2005;105(4):921–7.
17. Batt RE, Mitwally MF. Endometriosis from thelarche to midteens: pathogenesis and prognosis, prevention and pedagogy. J Pediatr Adolesc Gynecol 2003; 16(6):337–47.
18. Laufer MR, Goitein L, Bush M, et al. Prevalence of endometriosis in adolescent girls with chronic pelvic pain not responding to conventional therapy. J Pediatr Adolesc Gynecol 1997;10(4):199–202.
19. Redwine DB. Age-related evolution in color appearance of endometriosis. Fertil Steril 1987;48(6):1062–3.
20. Doyle JO, Missmer SA, Laufer MR. The effect of combined surgical-medical intervention on the progression of endometriosis in an adolescent and young adult population. J Pediatr Adolesc Gynecol 2009;22(4):257–63.
21. Lara-Torre E, Edwards CP, Perlman S, et al. Bone mineral density in adolescent females using depot medroxyprogesterone acetate. J Pediatr Adolesc Gynecol 2004;17(1):17–21.
22. Committee on Adolescent Health Care Long-Acting Reversible Contraception Working Group, The American College of Obstetricians and Gynecologists. Committee opinion no. 539: adolescents and long-acting reversible contraception: implants and intrauterine devices. Obstet Gynecol 2012;120(4):983–8.
23. Bayer LL, Hillard PJ. Use of levonorgestrel intrauterine system for medical indications in adolescents. J Adolesc Health 2013;52(Suppl 4):S54–8.
24. Trent M, Haggerty CL, Jennings JM, et al. Adverse adolescent reproductive health outcomes after pelvic inflammatory disease. Arch Pediatr Adolesc Med 2011; 165(1):49–54.

25. Lee V, Tobin JM, Foley E. Relationship of cervical ectopy to chlamydia infection in young women. J Fam Plann Reprod Health Care 2006;32(2):104–6.
26. Lenoir CD, Adler NE, Borzekowski DL, et al. What you don't know can hurt you: perceptions of sex-partner concurrency and partner-reported behavior. J Adolesc Health 2006;38(3):179–85.
27. Muolokwu E, Sanchez J, Bercaw JL, et al. The incidence and surgical management of paratubal cysts in a pediatric and adolescent population. J Pediatr Surg 2011;46(11):2161–3.
28. Amesse LS, Gibbs P, Hardy J, et al. Peritoneal inclusion cysts in adolescent females: a clinicopathological characterization of four cases. J Pediatr Adolesc Gynecol 2009;22(1):41–8.
29. Kanizsai B, Orley J, Szigetvári I, et al. Ovarian cysts in children and adolescents: their occurrence, behavior, and management. J Pediatr Adolesc Gynecol 1998; 11(2):85–8.
30. Spinelli C, Di Giacomo M, Cei M, et al. Functional ovarian lesions in children and adolescents: when to remove them. Gynecol Endocrinol 2009;25(5):294–8.
31. Kashima K, Yahata T, Fujita K, et al. Outcomes of fertility-sparing surgery for women of reproductive age with FIGO stage IC epithelial ovarian cancer. Int J Gynaecol Obstet 2013;121(1):53–5.
32. Rackow BW, Novi JM, Arya LA, et al. Interstitial cystitis is an etiology of chronic pelvic pain in young women. J Pediatr Adolesc Gynecol 2009;22(3):181–5.
33. Yoost JL, Hertweck SP, Loveless M. Diagnosis and treatment of interstitial cystitis in adolescents. J Pediatr Adolesc Gynecol 2012;25(3):162–71.
34. Huppert JS, Biro F, Lan D, et al. Urinary symptoms in adolescent females: STI or UTI? J Adolesc Health 2007;40(5):418–24.
35. Holland-Hall CM, Brown RT. Evaluation of the adolescent with chronic abdominal or pelvic pain. J Pediatr Adolesc Gynecol 2004;17(1):23–7.
36. Crabbe MM, Norwood SH, Robertson HD, et al. Recurrent and chronic appendicitis. Surg Gynecol Obstet 1986;163(1):11–3.
37. Seidman JD, Andersen DK, Ulrich S, et al. Recurrent abdominal pain due to chronic appendiceal disease. South Med J 1991;84(7):913–6.
38. Hawes AS, Whalen GF. Recurrent and chronic appendicitis: the other inflammatory conditions of the appendix. Am Surg 1994;60(3):217–9.
39. Chichom Mefire A, Tchounzou R, Kuwong PM, et al. Clinical, ultrasonographic, and pathologic characteristics of patients with chronic right-lower-quadrant abdominal pain that may benefit from appendectomy. World J Surg 2011;35(4): 723–30.
40. DeCou JM, Gauderer MW, Boyle JT, et al. Diagnostic laparoscopy with planned appendectomy: an integral step in the evaluation of unexplained right lower quadrant pain. Pediatr Surg Int 2004;20(2):123–6.
41. Lal AK, Weaver AL, Hopkins MR, et al. Laparoscopic appendectomy in women without identifiable pathology undergoing laparoscopy for chronic pelvic pain. JSLS 2013;17(1):82–7.
42. Schroeder B, Sanfilippo JS, Hertweck SP. Musculoskeletal pelvic pain in a pediatric and adolescent gynecology practice. J Pediatr Adolesc Gynecol 2000; 13(2):90.
43. Ling FW, Slocumb JC. Use of trigger point injections in chronic pelvic pain. Obstet Gynecol Clin North Am 1993;20(4):809–15.
44. Bedaiwy MA, Patterson B, Mahajan S. Prevalence of myofascial chronic pelvic pain and the effectiveness of pelvic floor physical therapy. J Reprod Med 2013; 58(11–12):504–10.

45. Song AH, Advincula AP. Adolescent chronic pelvic pain. J Pediatr Adolesc Gynecol 2005;18(6):371–7.
46. Greco CD. Management of adolescent chronic pelvic pain from endometriosis: a pain center perspective. J Pediatr Adolesc Gynecol 2003;16(Suppl 3):S17–9.
47. Kemper KJ, Sarah R, Silver-Highfield E, et al. On pins and needles? Pediatric pain patients' experience with acupuncture. Pediatrics 2000;105(4 Pt 2):941–7.
48. Walling MK, Reiter RC, O'Hara MW, et al. Abuse history and chronic pain in women: I. Prevalences of sexual abuse and physical abuse. Obstet Gynecol 1994;84(2):193–9.
49. Lampe A, Sölder E, Ennemoser A, et al. Chronic pelvic pain and previous sexual abuse. Obstet Gynecol 2000;96(6):929–33.
50. Lampe A, Doering S, Rumpold G, et al. Chronic pain syndromes and their relation to childhood abuse and stressful life events. J Psychosom Res 2003;54(4):361–7.
51. Elzevier HW, Voorham-van der Zalm PJ, Pelger RC. How reliable is a self-administered questionnaire in detecting sexual abuse: a retrospective study in patients with pelvic-floor complaints and a review of literature. J Sex Med 2007;4(4 Pt 1):956–63.
52. Alexander SC, Fortenberry JD, Pollak KI, et al. Sexuality talk during adolescent health maintenance visits. JAMA Pediatr 2014;168(2):163–9.
53. Boekeloo BO. Will you ask? Will they tell you? Are you ready to hear and respond?: barriers to physician-adolescent discussion about sexuality. JAMA Pediatr 2014;168(2):111–3.
54. Lindsetmo RO, Stulberg J. Chronic abdominal wall pain–a diagnostic challenge for the surgeon. Am J Surg 2009;198(1):129–34.
55. Hewitt G. Examining pediatric and adolescent gynecology patients. J Pediatr Adolesc Gynecol 2003;16(4):257–8.
56. Centers for Disease Control and Prevention. Recommendations for the laboratory-based detection of *Chlamydia trachomatis* and *Neisseria gonorrhoeae*–2014. MMWR Recomm Rep 2014;63(RR-02):1–19.
57. Hollman D, Coupey SM, Fox AS, et al. Screening for *Trichomonas vaginalis* in high-risk adolescent females with a new transcription-mediated nucleic acid amplification test (NAAT): associations with ethnicity, symptoms, and prior and current STIs. J Pediatr Adolesc Gynecol 2010;23(5):312–6.
58. Chapin K, Andrea S. APTIMA® Trichomonas vaginalis, a transcription-mediated amplification assay for detection of *Trichomonas vaginalis* in urogenital specimens. Expert Rev Mol Diagn 2011;11(7):679–88.

Surgical Evaluation and Treatment of the Patient with Chronic Pelvic Pain

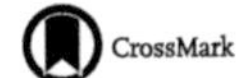

M. Brigid Holloran-Schwartz, MD

KEYWORDS

- Diagnostic laparoscopy and chronic pelvic pain
- Conscious laparoscopic pain mapping • Hysterectomy and chronic pain
- Presacral neurectomy • Laparoscopic uterine nerve ablation
- Adhesions and chronic pain

KEY POINTS

- Evaluation of the patient with chronic pelvic pain requires a detailed patient history, physical examination, ultrasonography, and pain diary.
- Nongynecologic sources of pelvic pain should be addressed concurrently. For example, constipation should be treated at the same time as cyclic dysmenorrhea.
- Diagnostic surgical evaluation should be offered to patients who have obvious abnormality on ultrasonography, in whom medical management has failed, or in whom the acuity of pain warrants an urgent diagnosis.
- Diagnostic laparoscopy and conscious laparoscopic pain mapping are useful in the surgical evaluation and treatment of chronic pelvic pain.
- Surgical treatments including excision of endometriosis, adhesiolysis, hysterectomy, and presacral neurectomy have been shown to provide relief to select patients. The possibility of persistent pain and new adhesion formation should be discussed with any patient considering surgery.

INTRODUCTION

Most gynecologists consider the definition of chronic pelvic pain to be pelvic pain of 6 months' duration. The subjective nature of pain makes studying pelvic pain with well-designed studies inherently difficult. Complicating matters, investigators of chronic pelvic pain often use variable definitions that include cyclic, intermittent, and noncyclic. In Practice Bulletin no. 51, the American College of Obstetricians and Gynecologists suggests one definition of chronic pelvic pain to be pain of 6 or more months' duration that localizes to the anatomic pelvis, anterior abdominal wall

---

The author has nothing to disclose.
Saint Louis University School of Medicine, Department of Obstetrics, Gynecology and Women's Health, 6420 Clayton Road, Suite 230, St Louis, MO 63117, USA
E-mail address: holloran@slu.edu

Obstet Gynecol Clin N Am 41 (2014) 357–369
http://dx.doi.org/10.1016/j.ogc.2014.05.003 **obgyn.theclinics.com**

at or below the umbilicus, the lumbosacral back, or the buttocks, and is of sufficient severity to cause functional disability or lead to medical care.[1] Approximately 15% to 20% of women aged 18 to 50 years have pelvic pain for longer than 1 year.[1] Despite this prevalence, there are many patients for whom the etiology is unclear.[2]

At the patient's initial consultation, medical and surgical options should be outlined (**Fig. 1**). Reviewing possible gynecologic, gastrointestinal, genitourinary, and musculoskeletal causes of pain will help the patient understand the importance of documenting alleviating and aggravating influences. Having the patient keep a pain diary for 3 months is helpful to further characterize the pain. Medical options, including nonsteroidal anti-inflammatory drugs, combined oral contraceptives, gonadotropin-releasing hormone agonists, and progesterone therapy may be offered as nonsurgical options, especially if there is a cyclical pattern.[3–8] If the patient suffers from predominantly gastrointestinal or genitourinary symptoms, referral should be made to these specialties to rule out other nongynecologic causes before diagnostic laparoscopy. If these patients return with persistent pain, especially after improvement in these systems, diagnostic laparoscopy may be offered. For the patient suffering from severe, disabling pain or the patient who declines or does not respond to medical therapy, a diagnostic laparoscopy may be offered. This article focuses on surgical interventions that may be offered for chronic pelvic pain, excluding endometriosis (addressed separately in the article by Yeung elsewhere in this issue).

DIAGNOSTIC SURGICAL PROCEDURES

Diagnostic Laparoscopy

The etiology of chronic pelvic pain is not always obvious after thorough history, physical examination, and imaging. Diagnostic laparoscopy can be offered in the absence of abnormality on physical examination or imaging, and has been increasingly used as

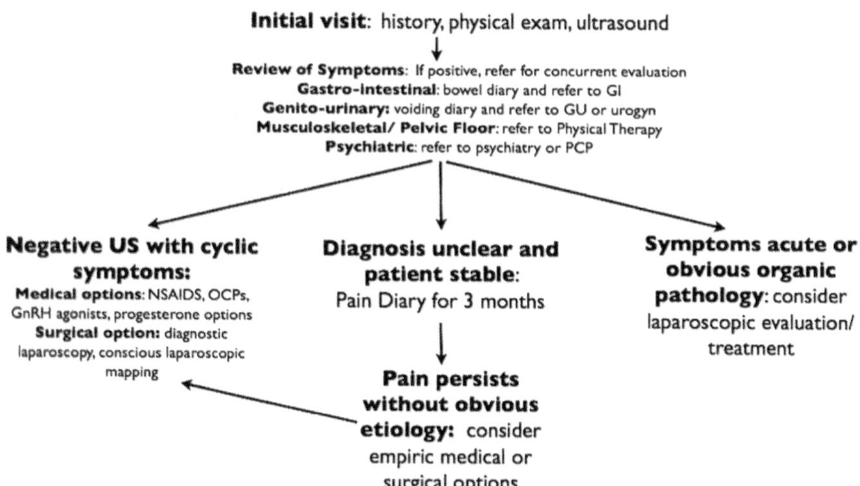
Evaluation of the Chronic Pelvic Pain
Initial visit: history, physical exam, ultrasound
Review of Symptoms: If positive, refer for concurrent evaluation
Gastro-intestinal: bowel diary and refer to GI
Genito-urinary: voiding diary and refer to GU or urogyn
Musculoskeletal/ Pelvic Floor: refer to Physical Therapy
Psychiatric: refer to psychiatry or PCP
Negative US with cyclic symptoms:
Medical options: NSAIDS, OCPs, GnRH agonists, progesterone options
Surgical option: diagnostic laparoscopy, conscious laparoscopic mapping
Diagnosis unclear and patient stable:
Pain Diary for 3 months
Symptoms acute or obvious organic pathology: consider laparoscopic evaluation/ treatment
Pain persists without obvious etiology: consider empiric medical or surgical options

Fig. 1. Pathways of chronic pelvic pain management. GI, gastrointestinal; GnRH, gonadotropin-releasing hormone; GU, genitourinary; NSAIDs, nonsteroidal anti-inflammatory drugs; OCPs, oral contraceptive pills; PCP, primary care physician.

a diagnostic tool, accounting for upward of 40% of laparoscopic procedures.[2] Despite its frequent use, there are no clear guidelines as to when this should be offered.

Diagnostic laparoscopy may be helpful in the evaluation of visceral sources of pain such as endometriosis, adhesions, ovarian masses, pelvic inflammatory disease, and malignancy.[9] Counseling patients about the risks, benefits, and expectations before surgery is important. Pelvic ultrasonography should be done preoperatively to allow discussion of obvious possible abnormality such as ovarian cysts. The patient should be consented for possible peritoneal biopsies and adhesiolysis. The goal of a laparoscopy is ideally to establish a diagnosis and provide surgical treatment in a single step. As the risk of adhesions increases with the total number of abdominal and pelvic surgeries, every surgery needs to be considered carefully.[2]

A thorough diagnostic laparoscopy usually involves at least a camera port and an accessory port to manipulate organs and assist with exposure. Additional ports may be needed if peritoneal biopsies or adhesiolysis is needed. Peritoneal biopsies of abnormal peritoneum are ideal for establishing a diagnosis, especially if endometriosis is suspected.[2] The patient should be counseled preoperatively on the possibility of not being able to identify any abnormality.

Conscious Laparoscopic Pain Mapping

Conscious laparoscopic pain mapping has been advocated by some as a useful tool in the evaluation of chronic pain.[10] The reasoning is that there is often poor correlation of the patient's symptoms and the findings at laparoscopy, even in the presence of obvious abnormality such as adhesive disease and endometriosis.[11,12] Nociceptive signals may originate from more than 1 organ, and adding the patient's own feedback can provide useful information to direct treatment options.

The procedure involves establishing laparoscopic access and then waking the patient sufficiently to allow her to comprehend questioning and provide feedback. This approach usually involves using short-acting anesthetic agents such as fentanyl and midazolam. A blunt probe is used to establish a "control area"; the surgeon may than proceed with palpating sites where the pain is suspected, such as the ovary or appendix. Care is taken to minimize other discomforts related to the surgical procedure itself, so lidocaine is used liberally at the site of the uterine manipulator and skin incisions, while lidocaine jelly is used with Foley catheter placement.[13] Possible outcomes of pain mapping should be discussed preoperatively with patients, including a possible plan of action (ie, appendectomy if there is pain in the appendix). If additional, more extensive surgery is needed, general anesthesia can be introduced and the procedure completed during the same operative event.[13]

Limitations are seen in those of higher body mass index who may require significant Trendelenburg and increased torque with instrument manipulation at port sites. Patients with anxiety, agoraphobia, claustrophobia, or a low pain tolerance may not able to tolerate the procedure.[10,14]

Patient responses have been described by Palter[13,15] and Palter and Olive,[16] who categorized these into 3 groups:

1. Focal pain elicited is greater in one area than in adjacent areas
2. Pain is stimulated not at all or at universally low levels of the pelvis
3. High levels of pain are generated throughout most of the pelvic structures probed

Well-designed studies are inherently difficult to design, as the patients and surgeons cannot be blinded and patient selection makes randomization difficult. Small case series have found successful pain mapping in 70% to 100% of patients.[9,16] The lack of more recent studies suggests a limitation on this being used as a global tool for general gynecologists.[10] At present, there remain no substantial data to confirm the accuracy or improved clinical outcomes with laparoscopic pain mapping.[1]

FINDINGS POTENTIALLY AMENABLE TO SURGICAL TREATMENT

Previous published studies of laparoscopic findings for the patient with chronic pelvic pain suggest that endometriosis is diagnosed in 33%, adhesive disease in 24%, and no visible abnormality in 35%.[2] This finding may differ in various parts of the world, as demonstrated by a recent publication from of Hyderabad, where pelvic tuberculosis was the most common disorder followed by endometriosis, pelvic inflammatory disease, and adhesions.[17] At the time of laparoscopy, careful attention and biopsy of all abnormally appearing peritoneum is helpful to confirm a histologic diagnosis, particularly given all the different appearances endometriosis can have.[9] In a well-designed study, Walter and colleagues[18] demonstrated the importance of biopsy confirmation of abnormality. In his study, the visual appearance of endometriosis, when compared with histologic diagnosis, had a positive predictive value of 45%, negative predictive value of 99%, sensitivity of 97%, and specificity of 77%. These values varied by location of anatomic site. Histologic confirmation is critical, especially if the patient's pain persists or recurs at a later time after surgery. Included in this review is a discussion of possible causes of pelvic pain that may be diagnosed or treated with laparoscopy, with the exclusion of endometriosis, which again is addressed by Yeung's article elsewhere in this issue.

Laparoscopy and Pelvic Adhesions

The incidence of pelvic adhesive disease is unknown, and its role in the patient with chronic pelvic pain is controversial. Pelvic adhesions can generally result from any peritoneal irritation or inflammation, such as previous pelvic surgery, endometriosis, appendicitis, or pelvic inflammatory disease. One of these is present in the history of approximately 50% of women with pelvic adhesions, with the remaining 50% having no such previous history.[19] Stovall and colleagues[19] found the incidence of pelvic adhesions to be between 27% and 60% in women undergoing laparoscopy for pelvic pain. Nerve fibers have been identified in the adhesions of patients with and without chronic pain.[20] However, most women with pelvic adhesions are asymptomatic.[9] Furthermore, the extent or location of pelvic adhesions does not always correlate with the location or severity of the pain.[2]

It is hypothesized that adhesions may be a source of pain when they cause distortion of the normal anatomic relationships and/or when activities cause stretching of the peritoneum or organ serosa at the adhesion's attachment site.[20] It may be a band, of variable density and vascularity, or a cohesive connection of surfaces without an intervening band. Bowel adhesions are a proposed cause of chronic pelvic pain, and a known cause of partial and complete small bowel obstruction, that tend to have more acute presentations. Physical examination and preoperative imaging are not always useful predictors of the presence or location of pelvic adhesions. Diagnostic laparoscopy is the procedure of choice for diagnosing pelvic adhesive disease. The goal of adhesiolysis is to restore normal anatomy, but it must be recognized that new adhesions may form after any surgical procedure (**Figs. 2** and **3**).

Meticulous surgical technique is critical, including minimizing tissue trauma, achieving optimal hemostasis, and minimizing the risk of infection. Unfortunately, despite these efforts new adhesions can be generated with each surgical procedure.[21,22] Surgeons may consider using adhesion-prevention adjuncts, although there is no ideal agent. Several anti-inflammatory drugs such as dexamethasone have been

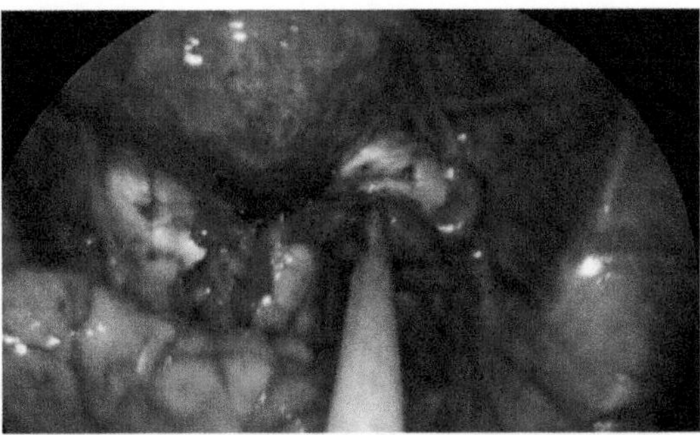

Fig. 2. An obliterated cul-de-sac in a patient with chronic pelvic pain and dense ovarian and bowel adhesions.

studied but have not proved to be effective.[23] In addition, there is insufficient evidence that peritoneal instillates such as normal saline or Ringer lactate, with or without heparin, prevent adhesions.[23] **Table 1** lists the advantages and disadvantages of the most effective adhesion-prevention barriers: Gore-Tex (Gore & Associates, Inc), Seprafilm (Genzyme), and Interceed (Ethicon Endo-Surgery).[21] One should avoid using oxidized regenerated cellulose (Interceed; Ethicon Endo-Surgery) in a patient for whom absolute hemostasis has not been achieved, as this may increase the risk of adhesions.[21]

The studies investigating laparoscopic adhesiolysis as a treatment for chronic pain are difficult to interpret collectively. Vrijland and colleagues[24] reviewed several observational studies with improvement ranging from 38% to 84%, but were limited by variable postoperative follow-up and pain-assessment tools. A randomized study assessing laparotomy alone versus laparotomy with adhesiolysis noted relief only for patients in whom dense bowel adhesions were noted.[25] Swank and colleagues[12] conducted a randomized controlled trial of diagnostic laparoscopy versus laparoscopic adhesiolysis in 100 participants (men and women) and found no difference in outcomes of pain or quality of life. At 1-year follow-up, 27% from each group continued to experience improved pain relief.

Laparoscopy and Ovarian Pathology

Ovarian cysts are thought to be an infrequent cause of chronic pelvic pain, accounting for only 3% of cases.[2] Most ovarian cysts are functional and asymptomatic, but can be a source of acute pain in the event of hemorrhage or torsion. If a functional ovarian cyst is suspected on ultrasonography in a stable patient, it generally can be followed with

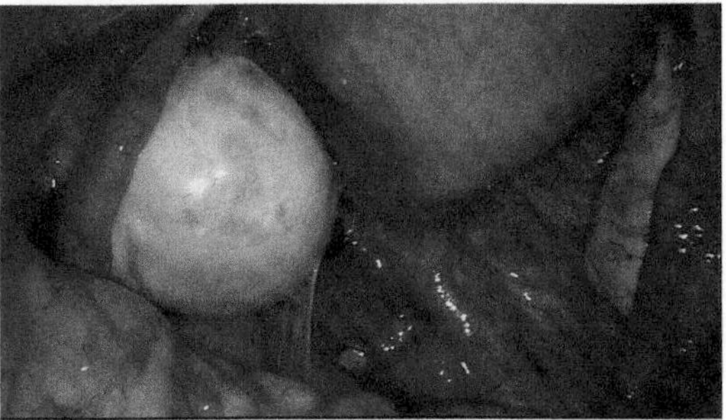

Fig. 3. Dense adhesions and an ovarian cyst limiting ovarian mobility.

Table 1
Advantages and disadvantages of adhesion prevention barriers

Adhesion Barrier	Advantages	Disadvantages
Polytetrafluoroethylene (Gore-Tex; W.L. Gore & Associates, Inc, Flagstaff, AZ)	Most effective adhesion barrier	Permanent material that needs to be sutured for security and later removed at subsequent surgery
Modified sodium hyaluronate/ carboxymethylcellulose (Seprafilm; Genzyme Corp, Boston, MA)	Effective at preventing adhesion formation in open surgery (myomectomies)	Lacking long-term studies. Not well studied laparoscopically
Oxidized regenerated cellulose (Interceed; Ethicon Endo-Surgery, Inc, Blue Ash, OH)	Effective at reducing pelvic adhesions during laparoscopy and laparotomy	May increase adhesion formation in the presence of blood

Data from Robertson D, Lefebvre G, Leyland N, et al. Adhesion prevention in gynaecological surgery. J Obstet Gynaecol Can 2010;32(6):598–608.

sonography and resolution documented after 1 to 2 cycles.[2] If recurrent, functional cyst formation is suspected as the source of intermittent cyclic pain, ovarian suppression with medical therapy, such as oral contraceptives, is usually successful.[2] The exception to this is ovarian endometriomas, which are most effectively treated with surgical cystectomy. Cystectomy is preferred over ovarian cyst drainage or cauterization of cyst lining, showing an improved reduction in pain and cyst recurrence (**Fig. 4**).[26]

Ovarian remnant syndrome is defined as the presence of ovarian tissue in a woman with a history of bilateral salpingo-oophorectomy that usually is the result of unintentional incomplete excision in the setting of severe adhesions, endometriosis, chronic pelvic inflammatory disease, or malignancy.[27] A premenopausal follicle-stimulating hormone value in a woman with a history of a bilateral salpingo-oophorectomy may help identify these patients. Various studies quote ovarian remnant syndrome as the

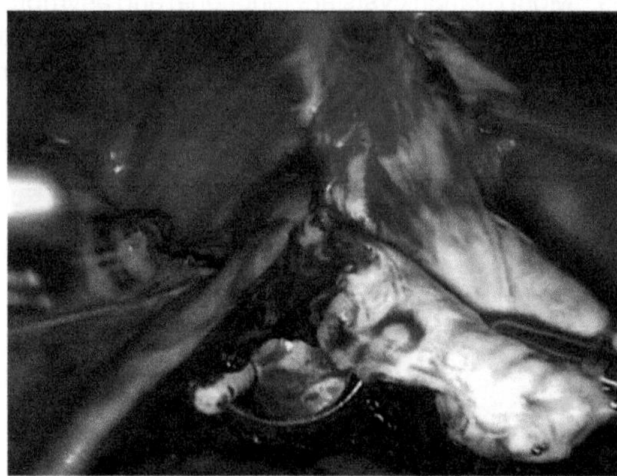

Fig. 4. Removal of ovarian cyst capsule using traction and countertraction, ligating small vessels.

cause of chronic pelvic pain in 18% to 26% of patients.[28,29] One study reported that in patients with chronic pelvic pain, a history of a bilateral salpingo-oophorectomy, and adnexal mass, ovarian remnant syndrome was identified in 76.5% of patients.[30] Management involves surgical excision through laparoscopy or laparotomy.[29,30]

Laparoscopy and Hernias

Hernias are found in only 1.6% to 6% of women with chronic pelvic pain.[31–33] Inguinal and femoral hernias may present with lateralizing chronic pelvic pain that may worsen with an upright position.[9] Sciatic hernias may radiate to the buttocks and posterior thigh.[34] A sciatic hernia is defined as a peritoneal sac with variable contents (fallopian tube or ovary) that protrudes through the greater or lesser sciatic foramen.[2] Inguinal, femoral, and sciatic hernias can be identified and repaired at laparoscopy.

Previous studies have described laparoscopic inguinal exploration and mesh placement in patients with chronic pelvic pain without a clinical hernia, hypothesizing that incarcerated fat in the inguinal canal may be a source of chronic pain.[35,36] Yong and colleagues[37] recently conducted a retrospective cohort study of empiric laparoscopic inguinal exploration and mesh placement in women with lateralizing chronic pelvic pain. Of 48 patients, 7 had an occult hernia they classified as a patent processus vaginalis, shown in **Fig. 5**.

Regardless of this finding, all 48 patients had inguinal exploration and mesh placement. Thirty-five percent had pain improvement regardless of the presence of an occult hernia. An additional 42% had initial improvement and later recurrence of pain (range of follow-up 73.2 $\pm$ 30.6 months). Patients with a positive Carnett test in the ipsilateral lower abdomen correlated with an improvement in pain. A positive Carnett test is defined as worsening in tenderness with abdominal wall flexion or contraction.[37] Additional studies are needed before this can be widely accepted as a treatment modality.

Laparoscopy and Pelvic Congestion Syndrome

Pelvic congestion syndrome is described as the presence of pelvic varices with subsequent venous stasis and congestion of the pelvic organs that results in chronic pelvic pain.[38] Laparoscopy has limited potential for the diagnosis of pelvic congestion syndrome, as the Trendelenburg position often results in the collapse of varicosities. Pelvic varicosities may be suspected if dilated veins (>8–10 mm in diameter) are seen in the reverse Trendelenburg position, but this has been shown to have a low sensitivity for diagnosis.[2,38] Venography, performed either transuterine or percutaneously, remains the gold standard for diagnosis of pelvic vascular congestion.[2,38]

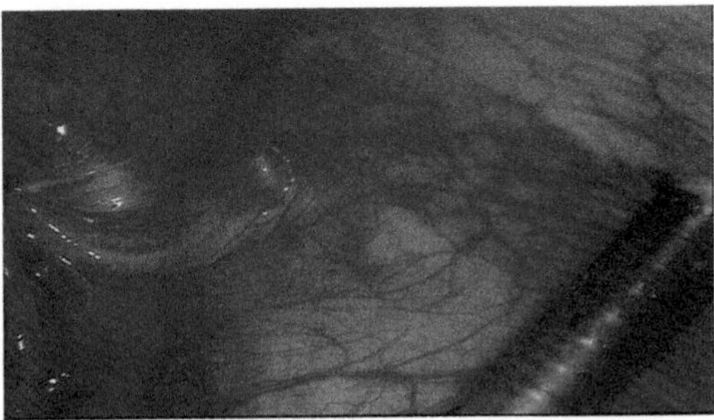

Fig. 5. A shallow peritoneal defect classified as a patent processus vaginalis or occult hernia.

Medical, surgical, and radiologic treatment options have been proposed for pelvic congestion syndrome. One randomized controlled trial by Soysal and colleagues[39] demonstrated improvement in symptoms with suppression of ovarian function with medroxyprogesterone acetate and goserelin. Hysterectomy, with and without bilateral salpingo-oophorectomy, has been shown to be effective in women in whom medical therapy has failed, but given the limited number of studies it should be used as a last resort.[40]

Radiographic embolotherapy has been shown to be as effective as hysterectomy in treating the symptoms of pelvic congestion syndrome.[41] Embolotherapy has the advantage of leaving no obvious scar, and can be performed on an outpatient basis. Several studies have documented the long-term effectiveness of this approach. Kim and colleagues[42] demonstrated efficacy in patients followed for 45 months. In addition, in a more recent study Laborda and colleagues[43] showed improvement in visual analog scores up to 5 years.

Laparoscopy and Endosalpingiosis

Endosalpingiosis is the presence of fallopian tube glandular epithelium in an ectopic location. It often resembles and is mistaken for endometriosis. Again this emphasizes the importance of excisional biopsies of abnormal peritoneum for tissue diagnosis in the management of the patient with chronic pain. The evidence supporting endosalpingiosis as a cause of chronic pelvic pain is primarily observational, based on a limited number of patients.[2] A recent study by Prentice and colleagues[44] found no significant relationship between endosalpingiosis, chronic pelvic pain, and infertility (**Fig. 6**).

PROCEDURES OFFERED FOR THE TREATMENT OF CHRONIC PELVIC PAIN

Hysterectomy

The role of hysterectomy in the treatment of idiopathic chronic pelvic pain is controversial. Approximately 12% of the 600,000 hysterectomies in the United States are done for reasons of chronic pelvic pain.[45] Before hysterectomy is considered, a multidisciplinary evaluation of any possible gastrointestinal, genitourinary, musculoskeletal, and/or psychiatric causes is necessary. When counseling patients considering hysterectomy for chronic pelvic pain, they should be informed that up to 40% of women will continue to have pain and 5% may have worsening symptoms.[46]

Lamvu[46] recently published a review on the role of hysterectomy in the treatment of chronic pelvic pain. She quoted a study by Stovall and colleagues[47] wherein patients who had failed other medical and surgical options underwent hysterectomy with a

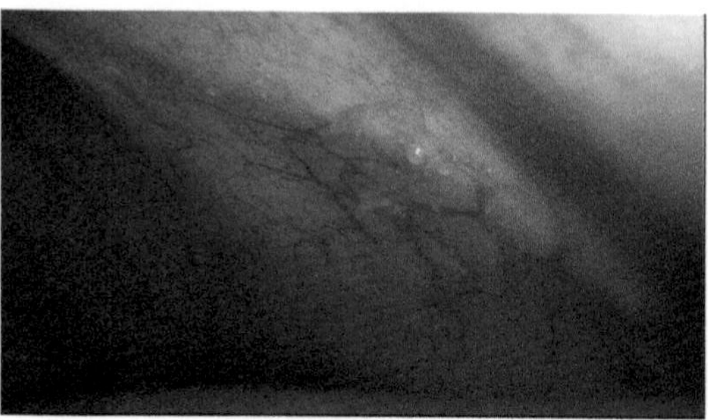

Fig. 6. Endosalpingiosis.

78% improvement rate. Of note, from this same study, 22% had persistence of pain even in the presence of histologic evidence of uterine disease.[47] Hillis and colleagues[48] found that in specific subsets of women, up to 40%, will continue to have pain. Specifically, women at increased risk for persistence were found to be younger than 30 years, uninsured, covered by Medicaid, had a history of pelvic inflammatory disease, and no identifiable abnormality at surgery. Lamvu[46] noted that these studies did not examine variables such as preexisting depression, anxiety, and history of abuse, which have been proved to be important in the modulation of long-term pain outcomes.

Hartmann and colleagues[49] looked at quality of life and sexual function after hysterectomy in patients with preoperative pain and depression over a 24-month period. Approximately 80% of patients were found to have improvement in pain, even in the presence of preexisting chronic pain, depression, or both after hysterectomy. Approximately 60% of patients reported improvement in pain with intercourse, although the frequency of intercourse remained unchanged.[49]

A 2006 retrospective cohort of 124 patients looked at patients with persistent chronic pain after hysterectomy and bilateral salpingo-oophorectomy. The most common histopathologic findings were adhesions (93%), adnexal remnants (32%), and endometriosis (18%).[28] Lamvu[46] concluded that all patients should have a thorough multidisciplinary evaluation before surgery to exclude other nonreproductive causes of pain before recommending hysterectomy with or without bilateral salpingo-oophorectomy. In addition, they should be counseled about the possible persistence of pain.

Laparoscopic Uterine Nerve Ablation

Laparoscopic uterine nerve ablation (LUNA) involves transection of the uterosacral ligaments at their insertion into the uterus with the purpose of interrupting the cervical sensory nerve fibers. It has been hypothesized that dividing these trunks may help women with dysmenorrhea.[50] A 2009 randomized controlled trial of 487 patients with chronic pelvic pain followed for 69 months, who had undergone laparoscopy with and without LUNA, found no difference in pain, dysmenorrhea, dyspareunia, or quality of life between the 2 arms.[50] Furthermore, a 2010 meta-analysis of randomized trials further analyzed available data and found no difference in improvement in pain between those who did or did not undergo LUNA.[51] At present, there is insufficient evidence to recommend LUNA (**Fig. 7**).

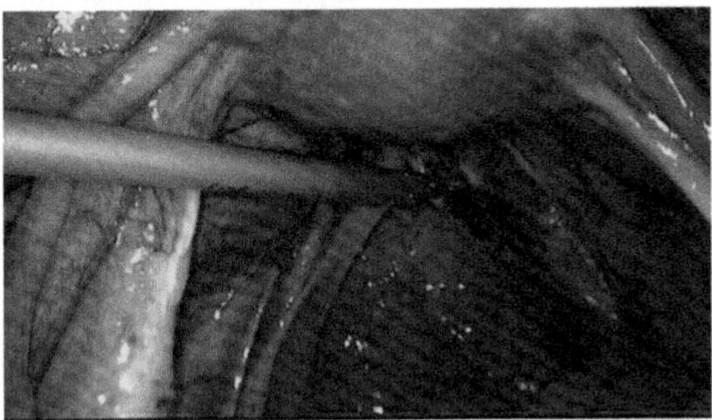

Fig. 7. The technique of laparoscopic uterine nerve ablation is performed by transecting both uterosacral ligaments at their attachment to the cervix. This photo shows transection of the right uterosacral ligament.

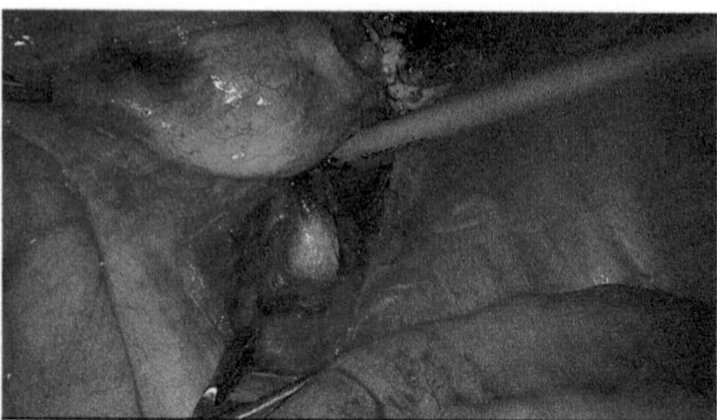

Fig. 8. Exposure of the presacral space for presacral neurectomy. The sacral promontory is noted at the tip of the laparoscopic grasper.

Presacral Neurectomy

Presacral neurectomy targets the superior hypogastric plexus (presacral nerves) that supply the cervix, uterus, and proximal fallopian tubes with afferent nociception. Surgical resection of this plexus has been shown to decrease dysmenorrhea unresponsive to other treatments.[1] It is significantly more effective than LUNA for the treatment of primary dysmenorrhea.[52] It is notable that central midline pelvic pain is much more responsive to presacral neurectomy than lateral pelvic pain, regardless of pathologic features.[1]

A recent 2012 retrospective analysis collected over 6 years demonstrated improvement in midline pain in 73% (22 of 30) of patients.[53]

Clinical trials in the early 1990s supported presacral neurectomy as an adjunct to conservative surgery for endometriosis, demonstrating additional midline pain relief associated with menses but not dyspareunia or nonmenstrual pain.[54,55] A more recent randomized controlled trial of 141 patients followed over 24 months demonstrated improvement in dysmenorrhea, dyspareunia, and quality of life in patients with endometriosis who underwent a concurrent presacral neurectomy at the time of conservative laparoscopic surgery over those who did not (**Fig. 8**).[56]

SUMMARY

It is important to characterize pelvic pain with a detailed patient history, physical examination, imaging, and a pain diary. Other possible nongynecologic causes must be addressed concurrently for optimal patient outcomes. Medical and surgical options should be outlined. Surgical therapy can be useful in patients with visceral sources of pain such as endometriosis, adhesions, ovarian disorder, hernias, pelvic inflammatory disease, and malignancy. In carefully selected patients, pelvic pain can be relieved with adhesiolysis, excision of endometriosis, hernia repair, hysterectomy, and presacral neurectomy. Before surgery the possibility of a negative laparoscopy, persistent postoperative pain, and new adhesion formation should be discussed.

REFERENCES

1. ACOG Practice Bulletin. Clinical management guidelines for obstetrician-gynecologists. No. 51, March 2004.
2. Howard FM. The role of laparoscopy in the chronic pelvic pain patient. Clin Obstet Gynecol 2003;46:749–66.

3. Owen PR. Prostaglandin synthetase inhibitions in the treatment of primary dysmenorrhea: outcome trials reviewed. Am J Obstet Gynecol 1984;148: 96–103.
4. Marjoribanks J, Proctor ML, Farquhar C. Nonsteroidal antiinflammatory drugs for primary dysmenorrhea [cochrane review]. In: Mary McLennan, Andrew Steele, Fah Che Leong, editors. The Cochrane library, Issue 4. Chichester (United Kingdom): John Wiley & Son, Ltd; 2003.
5. Proctor ML, Roberts H, Farquhar C. Combined oral contraceptive pill (OCP) as treatment for primary dysmenorrhea [cochrane review]. In: Mary McLennan, Andrew Steele, Fah Che Leong, editors. The Cochrane library, Issue 4. Chichester (United Kingdom): John Wiley & Son, Ltd; 2003.
6. Vercellini P, Aimi G, Panazza S, et al. A levonorgestrel-releasing intrauterine system for the treatment of dysmenorrhea associated with endometriosis. Fertil Steril 1999;72:505–8.
7. Telimaa S, Ronnberg L, Kauppila A. Placebo-controlled comparison of danazol and high-dose medroxyprogesterone acetate in the treatment of endometriosis after conservative surgery. Gynecol Endocrinol 1987;1:363–71.
8. Farquhar CM, Rogers V, Franks S, et al. A randomized controlled trial of medroxyprogesterone acetate and psychotherapy for the treatment of pelvic congestion. Br J Obstet Gynaecol 1989;96:1153–62.
9. Lamvu G, Tu F, As-Sanie S, et al. The role of laparoscopy in the diagnosis and treatment of conditions associated with chronic pelvic pain. Obstet Gynecol Clin North Am 2004;31:619–30.
10. Yunker A, Steege J. Practical guide to laparoscopic pain mapping. J Minim Invasive Gynecol 2010;17:8–11.
11. Fukaya T, Hoshiai H, Yajima A. Is pelvic endometriosis always associated with chronic pain? A retrospective study of 618 cases diagnosed by laparoscopy. Am J Obstet Gynecol 1993;169:719–22.
12. Swank DJ, Swank-Bordewijk SC, Hop WC, et al. Laparoscopic adhesiolysis in patients with chronic abdominal pain: a blinded randomized controlled multicenter trial. Lancet 2003;361:1247–51.
13. Palter S. Microlaparoscopy under local anesthesia and conscious pain mapping for the diagnosis and management of pelvic pain. Curr Opin Obstet Gynecol 1999;11:387–93.
14. Swanton A, Iyer L, Reginald PW. Diagnosis, treatment and follow up of women undergoing conscious pain mapping for chronic pelvic pain: a prospective cohort study. BJOG 2006;113:792–6.
15. Palter S. Office-based surgery and its role in the management of pelvic pain. In: Blackwell R, Olive D, editors. Chronic pelvic pain. New York: Springer; 1998. p. 167–82.
16. Palter S, Olive D. Office microlaparoscopy under local anesthesia for chronic pelvic pain. J Am Assoc Gynecol Laparosc 1996;3:359–64.
17. Baloch S, Khaskheli M, Malik A. Diagnostic laparoscopic findings in chronic pelvic pain. J Coll Physicians Surg Pak 2013;23(3):190–3.
18. Walter AJ, Hentz JG, Magtiboy PM, et al. Endometriosis: correlation between histologic and visual findings at laparoscopy. Am J Obstet Gynecol 2001;184: 1407–11.
19. Stovall TG, Elder RF, Ling FW. Predictors of pelvic adhesions. J Reprod Med 1989;34:345–8.
20. Hammoud A, Gago A, Diamond M. Adhesions in patients with chronic pelvic pain: a role for adhesiolysis. Fertil Steril 2004;82:1483–91.

21. Robertson D, Lefebvre G, Leyland N, et al. Adhesion prevention in gynaecological surgery. J Obstet Gynaecol Can 2010;32(6):598–608.
22. Neis KJ, Neis F. Chronic pelvic pain: cause, diagnosis and therapy from a gynaecologist's and an endoscopist's point of view. Gynecol Endocrinol 2009; 25(11):757–61.
23. Pfeifer S, Lobo R, Goldberg J, et al, Practice Committee of American Society for Reproductive Medicine in collaboration with Society of Reproductive Surgeons. Pathogenesis, consequences and control of peritoneal adhesions in gynecologic surgery: a committee opinion. Fertil Steril 2013;99(6):1550–5.
24. Vrijland WW, Jeekel J, Geldor HJ, et al. Abdominal adhesions: intestinal obstruction, pain, and infertility. Surg Endosc 2003;17(7):1017–22.
25. Peters AA, Trimbos-Kemper GC, Admiraal C, et al. A randomized clinical trial on the benefits of adhesiolysis in patients with intaperitoneal adhesions and chronic pelvic pain. BJOG 1992;99:59–62.
26. Yoshida S, Harada T, Iwabe T, et al. Laparoscopic surgery for the management of ovarian endometrioma. Gynecol Obstet Invest 2002;54(Suppl 1): 24–7.
27. Shemwell RW, Weed JC. Ovarian remnant syndrome. Obstet Gynecol 1970;36: 299–300.
28. Behera M, Vilos G, Hollett-Caines J, et al. Laparoscopic findings, histopathologic evaluation, and clinical outcomes in women with chronic pelvic pain after hysterectomy and bilateral salpingo-oophorectomy. J Minim Invasive Gynecol 2006;13: 431–5.
29. Abu-Rafeh B, Vilos GA, Misra M. Frequency and laparoscopic management of ovarian remnant syndrome. J Am Assoc Gynecol Laparosc 2003;10:33–7.
30. Senapati S, Advincula AP. Adnexal remnant syndrome: a new paradigm. J Am Assoc Gynecol Laparosc 2005;12:S7.
31. Banerjee S, Farrell RJ, Lembo T. Gastroenterological causes of pelvic pain. World J Urol 2001;19:166–72.
32. Carter JE. Combined hysteroscopic and laparoscopic findings in patients with chronic pelvic pain. J Am Assoc Gynecol Laparosc 1994;2:43–7.
33. Demco LA. Effect on negative laparoscopy rate in chronic pelvic pain patients using patient assisted laparoscopy. JSLS 1997;1:319–21.
34. Miklos JR, O'Reilly MJ, Saye WB. Sciatic hernia as a cause of chronic pelvic pain in women. Obstet Gynecol 1998;91:998–1001.
35. Metzger DA. Hernias in women: uncommon or unrecognized? Laparoscopy Today 2004;3(1):8–10.
36. Janicki TI, Onders R, Blood BJ, et al. Occult inguinal hernias in women with chronic pelvic pain. J Am Assoc Gynecol Laparosc 2001;8(Suppl 3):S28.
37. Yong P, Williams C, Allaire C. Laparoscopic inguinal exploration and mesh placement for chronic pelvic pain. JSLS 2013;17:74–81.
38. Liddle AD, Davies AH. Pelvic congestion syndrome: chronic pelvic pain caused by ovarian and internal iliac varices. Phlebology 2007;22(3):100–4.
39. Soysal ME, Soysal S, Vicdan K, et al. A randomised controlled trial of goserelin and medroxyprogesterone acetate in the treatment of pelvic congestion. Humanit Rep 2001;16:931–9.
40. Beard RW, Kennedy RG, Gangar KF, et al. Bilateral oophorectomy and hysterectomy in the treatment of intractable pelvic pain associated with pelvic congestion. Br J Obstet Gynaecol 1991;98:988–92.
41. Chung MH, Huh CY. Comparison of treatments for pelvic congestion syndrome. Tohoku J Exp Med 2003;201:131–8.

42. Kim HS, Malhotra AD, Rowe PC, et al. Embolotherapy for pelvic congestion syndrome: long-term results. J Vasc Interv Radiol 2006;17(2 Pt 1):289–97.
43. Laborda A, Medrano J, de Blas I, et al. Endovascular treatment of pelvic vascular congestion syndrome: visual analog score (VAS) long term follow up clinical evaluation in 202 patients. Cardiovasc Intervent Radiol 2013;36(4): 1006–14. http://dx.doi.org/10.1007/s00270-013-0586-2.
44. Prentice L, Stewart A, Mohiuddin S, et al. What is endosalpingiosis? Fertil Steril 2012;98(4):942–7.
45. We JM, Wechter ME, Geller EJ, et al. Hysterectomy rates in the United States, 2003. Obstet Gynecol 2007;110:1091–5.
46. Lamvu G. Role of hysterectomy in the treatment of chronic pelvic pain. Obstet Gynecol 2011;117:1175–8.
47. Stovall TG, Ling FW, Crawford DA. Hysterectomy for chronic pelvic pain of presumed uterine etiology. Obstet Gynecol 2004;104:701–9.
48. Hillis SD, Marchbanks PA, Peterson HB. The effectiveness of hysterectomy for chronic pelvic pain. Obstet Gynecol 1995;86:941–5.
49. Hartmann KE, Ma C, Lamvu GM, et al. Quality of life and sexual function after hysterectomy in women with preoperative pain and depression. Obstet Gynecol 2004;104:701–9.
50. Daniels J, Gray R, Hills RK, et al. Laparoscopic uterine nerve ablation for alleviating chronic pelvic pain: a randomized controlled trial. JAMA 2009;302(9): 955–61.
51. Daniels JP, Middleton L, Xiong T, et al. Individual patient data meta-analysis of randomized evidence to assess the effectiveness of laparoscopic uterine nerve ablation in patients with chronic pelvic pain. Hum Reprod Update 2010;16(6): 568–76.
52. Chen FP, Chang SD, Chu KK, et al. Comparison of laparoscopic presacral neurectomy and laparoscopic uterine nerve ablation for primary dysmenorrhea. J Reprod Med 1996;41:463–6.
53. Kapetanakis V, Jacob K, Klauschie J, et al. Robotic presacral neurectomy - technique and results. Int J Med Robot 2012;8:73–6.
54. Canadiani GB, Fedele L, Vercillini P, et al. Presacral neurectomy for the treatment of pelvic pain associated with endometriosis: a controlled study. Am J Obstet Gynecol 1992;167:100–3.
55. Tjaden B, Schlaff WD, Kimball A, et al. The efficacy of presacral neurectomy for the relief of midline dysmenorrhea. Obstet Gynecol 1990;76:89–91.
56. Zullo F, Palomba S, Zupi E, et al. Long-term effectiveness of presacral neurectomy for the treatment of severe dysmenorrhea due to endometriosis. J Am Assoc Gynecol Laparosc 2004;11:23–8.

The Laparoscopic Management of Endometriosis in Patients with Pelvic Pain

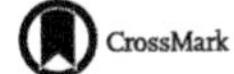

Patrick Yeung Jr, MD

KEYWORDS

• Endometriosis • Excision surgery • Laser surgery • Diagnostic imaging • Pelvic pain • Recurrence

KEY POINTS

- Diagnostic laparoscopy is indicated for women whose quality of life is significantly affected, for whom hormonal suppression has failed (or is contraindicated), or who desire fertility.
- Transvaginal ultrasonographic imaging (which may include evaluation for deep endometriosis) can aid in surgical planning.
- Optimal excision or removal of disease is the best way to reduce recurrence rates, and may also be a way to conserve normal ovaries and avoid surgical menopause, even when hysterectomy or definitive therapy is indicated.
- Early diagnosis and treatment may be the best way to prevent the development of extensive disease and, perhaps, to preserve fertility.

Video of ureterolysis accompanies this article at http://www.obgyn.theclinics.com/

INTRODUCTION

Endometriosis is estimated to be present in 1 of every 10 women.[1,2] It is a condition whereby endometrial glands and stroma (normally found within the endometrial cavity and shed during the menstrual period) are found outside the uterine cavity. Endometriosis is an underdiagnosed and undertreated problem, and multiple studies have shown that it can take an average of up to 12 years to diagnose (especially in teenagers) from the time of onset of symptoms to the diagnosis at laparoscopy.[3–6] This delay in diagnosis can contribute to impaired quality of life and may have implications for fertility.[7–9]

Center for Endometriosis, Division of Minimally Invasive Gynecologic Surgery, Department of Obstetrics, Gynecology & Women's Health, Saint Louis University, 6420 Clayton Road, Suite 290, St Louis, MO 63117, USA
E-mail address: pyeung1@slu.edu

Obstet Gynecol Clin N Am 41 (2014) 371–383
http://dx.doi.org/10.1016/j.ogc.2014.05.002

Laparoscopy is the gold standard for the diagnosis of endometriosis, by visualization of implants characteristic of endometriosis or, better still, by histology of excised lesions.[10] Laparoscopy is also the preferred route for treatment (when possible) of endometriosis because laparoscopy affords the benefits of magnification, illumination, and high-definition optics to better visualize the disease.

Although there is no cure for endometriosis, optimal laparoscopic management can benefit patients with pain (and improve fertility) and improve their quality of life.[11–13] Patients with endometriosis might benefit from early diagnosis and laparoscopic management, before progression of the disease, and providers should know when to operate and when to refer these patients.[8]

ENDOMETRIOSIS AND PAIN

Endometriosis is known to be associated with pain, and should be thought of as part of a comprehensive evaluation for pain.[9] During the adolescent period at least 75% of patients who failed medical treatment were found to have endometriosis.[7] Some algorithms recommend a diagnostic laparoscopy later in the evaluation after all other causes of pain have been ruled out or treated, including interstitial cystitis, vaginismus or myofascial pain, and pudendal neuralgia. Others recommend diagnostic laparoscopy sooner because endometriosis, unlike other causes of pain, can affect fertility, and surgical management for endometriosis may improve or preserve fertility.[9,14]

Although it is known that endometriosis and pain are associated, the exact causal relationship is not clear. Of note, the extent of disease (based on the most widely used revised American Society of Reproductive Medicine [r-ASRM] classification system[15]) does not correlate well with the severity of symptoms.[16] The way that endometriosis is currently classified is based on extent of disease, the presence of endometriomas, and adnexal or cul-de-sac adhesions. Deep endometriosis (or deep infiltrating endometriosis [DIE]) is not a part of the current classification system. However, there is evidence to show that the location of deep endometriosis has some correlation to the location of pain,[17] whereas the location of superficial endometriosis does not.[18] Newer classification systems are being developed to include DIE.[19]

HORMONAL VERSUS SURGICAL MANAGEMENT

Hormonal suppression is often recommended as first-line treatment for pain thought to arise from endometriosis.[10] Hormonal suppression can improve symptoms such as pelvic pain and dysmenorrhea. Empiric therapy with hormonal suppression, including a gonodotropin-releasing hormone agonist (GnRHa) or birth control pills, is often used to control symptoms, as a form of diagnostic trial, and to prevent progression of disease. However, a response to empiric therapy (meaning improvement in symptoms), for example, with a GnRHa, is not diagnostic for the presence of endometriosis.[10] Failure of pain to respond adequately to hormonal suppression should be investigated further for endometriosis.

Hormone suppression may do little to prevent recurrence or progression of the actual disease. A study of 90 patients by Doyle and colleagues[20] in 2009 showed that hormonal suppression given after surgery worsened (10%) or did not change staging or extent of the disease (70%) in 4 of every 5 women. Moreover, studies have shown that the need for hormonal suppression to control pain in earlier years may be a marker for more advanced disease. Studies by Chapron and colleagues[21–23] in 2011 showed that patients with severe endometriosis, when questioned about their adolescent history, had greater school absenteeism and an earlier or extended need for hormonal suppression to control pain in the adolescent years.

Finally, hormonal suppression does not improve fertility, neither while the patient is on suppression nor in the future.[24,25]

DIAGNOSIS

History and Evaluation

Symptoms characteristic of endometriosis include the following: dysmenorrhea, chronic pelvic pain (more than 3 months of pelvic pain outside the menstrual period, between the umbilicus and the thighs), deep dyspareunia, period-related dyschezia, and period-related dysuria.[10] Chronic pelvic pain has many different potential causes and is often multifactorial. Causes of chronic pelvic pain include endometriosis, pelvic inflammatory disease, interstitial cystitis, urinary tract infection, myofascial pain or vaginismus, and irritable bowel syndrome, to name a few.[26] A thorough evaluation and testing of the causes of chronic pain should be performed as directed by the history. Moreover, chronic pelvic pain can lead to centralization or sensitization to pain, which may need to be addressed. Under such circumstances the brain is sensitized to feeling pain even when the source of pain is treated or diminished.[27] A multimodal team approach is often the best way to treat chronic pelvic pain. Within the evaluation for chronic pelvic pain, endometriosis should be especially addressed if fertility or future fertility is desired.[28]

Indications for Laparoscopy

Providers who care for women should have a high index of suspicion for endometriosis when symptoms affect activities of daily living or quality of life. Examples include pelvic pain or dysmenorrhea that leads to absenteeism from school or work, deep dyspareunia that prohibits intercourse, or the need for narcotics to deal with pelvic pain.[12] In the adolescent population in particular, patients who have chronic pelvic pain but whose symptoms fail to improve with hormonal suppression have a very high prevalence of endometriosis. Experts have recommended that expectant management is inappropriate in patients with a visual analog scale score of greater than 7 or in patients with a poor quality of life as subjectively assessed by the patient.[29]

Infertility is another reason to perform laparoscopy for endometriosis. Historically, all patients with infertility have received a routine laparoscopy for evaluation of endometriosis given the known association of endometriosis with infertility. Current recommendations for laparoscopy because of fertility concerns include: age younger than 30 years; when in vitro fertilization (IVF) is not an option; or when a patient has failed 2 attempts at IVF.[28] The laparoscopic management of endometriosis has been shown to improve both pain[30] and fertility outcomes.[13,31] In a recent study by Lee and colleagues,[32] 42% of patients (with endometriosis ranging from stages I to IV) conceived successfully without hormonal treatment or artificial reproductive technologies within a year after surgery. In another study by Darai and colleagues[33] in 2005, pregnancy rates for a cohort of 34 women requiring colorectal bowel resection for advanced disease was 45% within 24 months.

The Potential Benefit of Early Diagnosis and Treatment of Endometriosis

Endometriosis is thought to be a progressive disease, although not in all cases.[8,34] Thus extensive or deep disease can arise from superficial disease. Some have touted the benefits of diagnosing and treating endometriosis earlier in the disease process, even in adolescence, which could improve lifelong pain and quality of life, and reduce the rate of progression to more advanced disease.[13] Early intervention and optimal removal of disease, by reducing the rate of recurrence or progression, has the potential to improve or preserve downstream fertility,[12] although this has to be systematically studied.

Preoperative Examination

The goal of surgery should be to "see and treat" laparoscopy when possible.[35] That is, at laparoscopy the disease is fully identified and optimally treated at the same time. The best way to achieve this is with thorough preoperative planning that includes history, physical examination, and preoperative imaging, usually transvaginal ultrasonography (TVUS). A physical examination should include assessment of the uterosacral ligaments (thickening, shortening, nodularity), mobility of the uterus and adnexa, adnexal masses, and a rectovaginal examination for cul-de-sac nodularity. Deep disease may be able to be diagnosed or suspected preoperatively, and ideally managed at surgery in a multidisciplinary fashion if necessary.[36] A history of dyschezia may increase suspicion for deep disease. A fixed or immobile uterus, or cul-de-sac nodularity, would imply an obliterated cul-de-sac or deep endometriosis.

Preoperative Imaging

TVUS is the imaging modality of choice for the assessment of suspected endometriomas or deep endometriosis. TVUS is an excellent imaging modality for female reproductive organs, and can be performed in the gynecologist office setting, although it is fairly operator-dependent.[10] With proper training and experience in specialized centers, TVUS with bowel preparation (TVUS-BP), whereby the distal bowel has been emptied by an enema, has been shown to be as accurate as pelvic magnetic resonance imaging in diagnosing deep endometriosis in the posterior cul-de-sac.[37–40]

Preoperative ultrasonography may indicate deep disease directly, or indirectly if an endometrioma larger than 8 cm or bilateral endometriomas are suspected.[41,42] In 2010 Goncalves and colleagues,[37] in a study involving 194 patients, showed the ability of TVUS-BP to predict the number of lesions in cases of deep endometriosis with a sensitivity and specificity of 97% and 100%, respectively (for a single bowel nodule), and with a positive predictive value (PPV) and negative predictive value (NPV) of 100% and 98%, respectively. Regarding the diagnosis of infiltration of the submucosal/mucosal layer, TVUS-BP had a sensitivity of 83%, specificity 94%, PPV 77%, and NPV 96%. Clearly this type of accurate imaging would be invaluable in helping to define the surgical strategy.

If the surgeon or center is not able to manage deep endometriosis suspected before surgery or discovered at the time of surgery, the patient should be referred to a surgeon or center that is able to manage deep or extensive endometriosis.[13,43]

SURGICAL TECHNIQUES

The goals of laparoscopic surgery for endometriosis are: optimal removal or treatment of all visible and deep disease; restoration and preservation of anatomy and function; and adhesion prevention.[29] Pelvic pain and fertility can be improved with surgical intervention.[30,31]

Near-Contact Laparoscopy

For early or mild forms of endometriosis (r-ASRM Stage 1–2), optimal excision depends first on recognizing endometriosis in all of its forms.[11] The most common way to diagnose endometriosis is to visualize typical implants that have a "powder-burn" appearance. However, a histologic diagnosis is more accurate, especially when the lesions have a more atypical or subtle appearance. Atypical lesions include "red flame" lesions, white fibrotic lesions, vesicular or miliary lesions, and retraction pockets (sometimes called Allen-Masterson pockets) (**Figs. 1** and **2**).[44] Careful and systematic near-contact laparoscopy should be used to find all lesions suspicious for endometriosis (**Fig. 3**).[44]

Removal of Deep Disease

For more advanced (or deep) endometriosis (r-ASRM Stage 2–4), optimal excision depends on not just recognition of peritoneal or superficial disease, but on recognition of deep disease and restoration of anatomy.[45] Surgery in these cases often includes bilateral ureterolysis, cystectomy, adhesiolysis, and enterolysis, and opening of an obliterated cul-de-sac or "frozen" pelvis. Of note, adhesions distort not just anatomy but also visualization of endometriosis, so adhesiolysis alone is insufficient to achieve an optimal surgical result. Once adhesions have been reduced, excision of the peritoneum or deep disease must occur for proper treatment of endometriosis (**Fig. 4**). It has been suggested that surgery for ovarian endometriosis alone is insufficient treatment.[42,46] Evidence shows that treatment of deep endometriosis, including bowel endometriosis and ovarian endometriomas, has been shown to benefit both pain and pregnancy outcomes,[13] with low recurrence rates.[47,48] Some have recommended that centers of excellence be created to manage difficult or challenging cases of endometriosis.[49]

Excision Versus Ablation

There is an ongoing debate about the best surgical method to treat endometriosis. Published comparative studies[50,51] do not account for surgical experience, nor of the presence of deep endometriosis. There are several surgical scenarios in which excision (removing the disease whereby a specimen is produced and sent to histology) is intuitively superior to ablation (destruction of the disease with energy without a specimen being produced). Such situations would include: deep endometriosis (whereby ablation would just treat the "tip of the iceberg"); ovarian endometriomas (which can be thought of as a form of deep endometriosis, see later discussion); endometriosis over a vital organ such as the bladder, bowel, or ureter; a patch of endometriosis or an area of peritoneum after adhesiolysis; a retraction pocket of peritoneum often caused by endometriosis. It is sometimes difficult to know when a superficial lesion involves deeper tissue, and excision has been advocated by some investigators for all cases of endometriosis.[12,52]

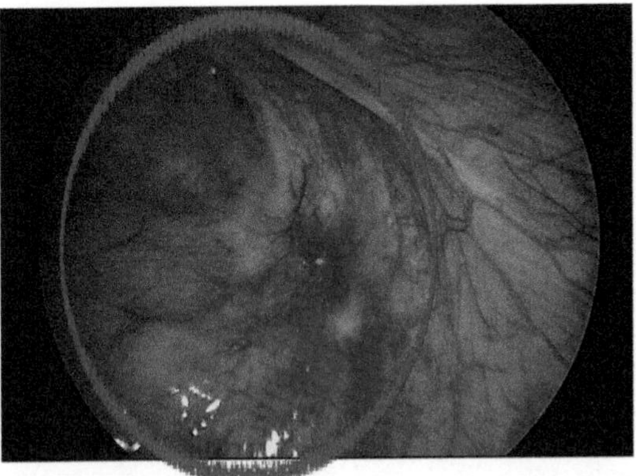

Fig. 1. Atypical and subtle phenotype of adolescent endometriosis as widespread brown lesions.

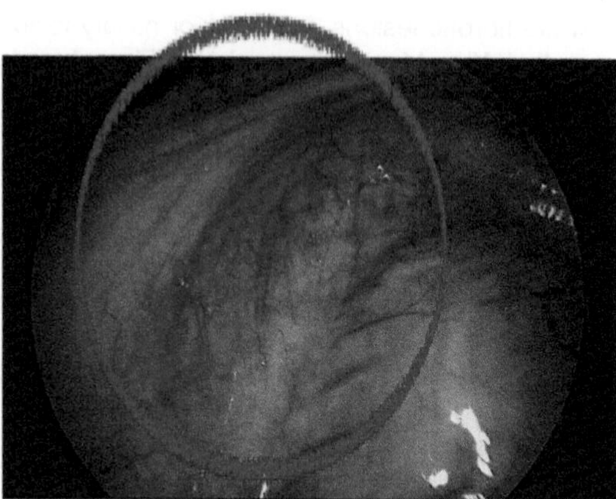

Fig. 2. Atypical and subtle phenotype of adolescent endometriosis as widespread vesicular or miliary lesions.

Energy Sources

Energy sources that have been used (for excision or ablation) include monopolar scissors, "cold" scissors, ultrasonic energy (harmonic scalpel), and lasers (potassium titanyl phosphate or KTP, neodymium-doped yttrium aluminum garnet or Nd:YAG, carbon dioxide or CO_2). The type of energy used is not as important as understanding the energy and being able to use the energy source to achieve optimal surgical treatment of the disease. For example, with monopolar energy, because the energy arcs from the tip of the instrument to the tissue (and then through the body to ground), the type of current and the presenting surface area (power density) of the instrument are important variables. It is recommended with monopolar energy (35–40 W and sometimes higher) to minimize the surface area of the presenting tip (using the utmost tip of the scissors) and to use cut current to increase cutting precision and reduce lateral thermal injury. With the free-beam CO_2 laser, higher power (in the range of 12–15 W) can increase the precision of the laser as a cutting instrument, although one must be careful not to let the laser dwell in one place over vital structures. Safe practice, knowledge of the energy, and proper training are important for whichever energy source is used.

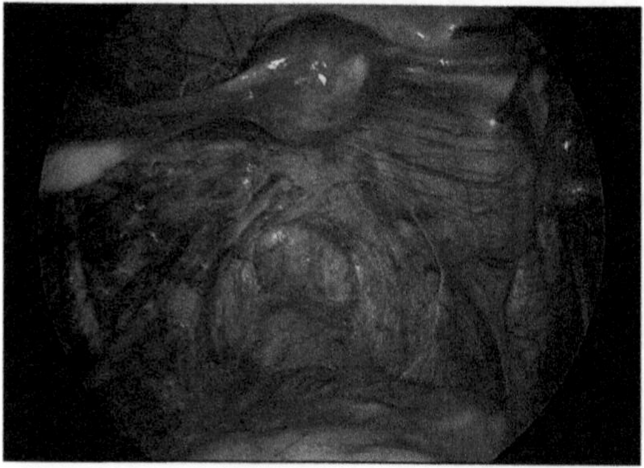

Fig. 3. The goal of endometriosis surgery is optimal excision of all visible lesions, both typical and atypical, with minimal char and good hemostasis.

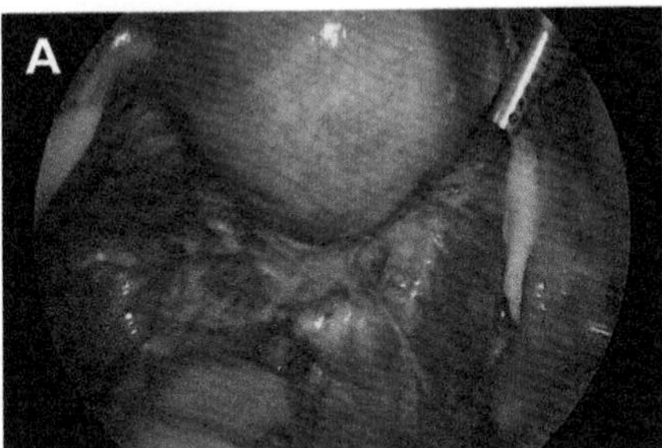

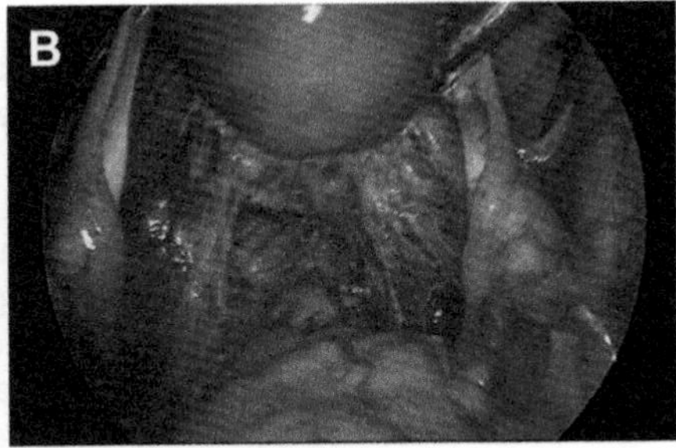

Fig. 4. (*A, B*) The goal of surgery for endometriosis with an obliterated cul-de-sac is restoration of anatomy and excision of visible or deep disease.

Treating Endometriomas

Evidence supports cystectomy (removal of the entire cyst wall) over incision and drainage for the treatment of ovarian endometriomas or "chocolate cysts," pain, recurrence, and fertility.[53] In cases where a cycle-day 3 follicle-stimulating hormone levels and antimullerian hormone (AMH) levels suggest reduced ovarian reserve, patients should be given an opportunity to harvest ova for future use if desired. Cystectomy has not been shown to negatively affect controlled hyperstimulation results.[54] Cystectomy has been shown to reduce AMH levels,[55,56] although it would seem that good surgical technique in finding the true plane between the cyst wall and the normal ovarian tissue is important.[57] In addition, it is unclear whether the presence of an untreated endometrioma is also associated with a similar decline in AMH.[58] Overall, most fertility specialists (95%) would offer cystectomy for endometriomas in patients for whom IVF is not an option, or for larger endometriomas (>3 cm) for patients undergoing IVF.[59]

Other Techniques

Ureterolysis is an important technique that should be used when lesions are found over the ureter. Gynecologists who treat endometriosis should be familiar and comfortable with performing ureterolysis when appropriate. Ureterolysis involves freeing the ureter off the peritoneum, usually by sweeping parallel to the direction of the ureter on the medial side (Video 1). Bilateral ureterolysis is also an essential step when approaching an obliterated cul-de-sac.

Exploration and dissection of the retroperitoneal space and ureterolysis are important techniques for any surgeon treating advanced endometriosis or deep disease. Knowledge of the retroperitoneal anatomy, the course of the ureter, and how to control bleeding by procedures such as hypogastric artery or uterine artery ligations will aid in excising deep pelvic endometriosis. Treatment of an obliterated cul-de-sac requires a systematic approach to restoring the anatomy and removing the disease, which usually involves cystectomy, bilateral ureterolysis, and a lateral to medial approach to release the bowel from the retrocervical or rectovaginal space. Vignali and colleagues[48] showed that surgical completeness of removal of deep disease will affect the rate of recurrence of endometriosis.

Preoperative Bowel Preparation

Preoperative bowel preparation has traditionally been used for diagnostic/operative laparoscopy for endometriosis, especially in cases when bowel endometriosis, deep endometriosis, or an obliterated cul-de-sac is suspected. Systematic reviews no longer recommend preoperative bowel preparation for gynecologic surgery, because it has not been shown to decrease the risk of bowel repair leakage or the need for colostomy.[60,61] That said, it is important to discuss the use of preoperative bowel preparation with the colorectal or general surgeon participating in the patient's care.

Definitive Surgery

Many consider definitive surgery for endometriosis to be total hysterectomy and bilateral salpingo-oophorectomy. The reasoning is to remove the uterus and thus the risk of adenomyosis (and, because menstruation is often painful, even without a pathologic diagnosis of adenomyosis), and to cause a surgical menopause to remove the stimulation of endometriosis left in the pelvis. The problem with this approach is that the actual disease remains and can still cause symptoms (especially deep endometriosis), and the benefits of ovarian hormone production have been lost, including cardiovascular and bone health. Another surgical approach that should be considered, especially in younger women who have completed childbearing, is to optimally remove the endometriosis and the uterus (again to reduce the risk of adenomyosis) with the fallopian tubes (not needed without the uterus and to reduce the risk of ovarian cancer[62]), but to conserve at least one, or both, ovaries.

Recurrence Rates

Recurrence rates of actual disease depend on the technique used, especially for deep endometriosis. Rates of recurrence (or persistence) of endometriosis after ablation are approximately 20% to 50% in 2 years[63,64] (approaching 50% by 5 years[65]), but as low as 0% at 2 years after optimal excision.[11] Of note, adding hormonal suppression after surgery does not further reduce the rate of actual recurrence of disease beyond the benefit of what is done at surgery, as noted by Doyle and colleagues[20] (see earlier discussion). Recurrence of pain does not necessarily indicate recurrence or persistence of endometriosis. In particular, when optimal endometriosis surgery has been achieved, other causes of pain should be evaluated before repeat surgery.

Recurrence rates after conservative surgery, even for advanced or deep disease, can be low (<10% in 3 years),[48] which depends on the surgical completeness of removing the disease. It has been suggested that extensive endometriosis can be avoided by early diagnosis and intervention in the disease, even in the adolescent years.[11,13]

Adhesion Prevention

Adhesion prevention is very important for reducing pain, avoiding complications such as bowel obstruction,[66] and preserving fertility.[67] Some have criticized excision

Table 1
Summary of fluid agents studied for the prevention of adhesions

Company	Product	Notes
—	Hyaluronic acid	Fluids that contain this product may decrease scar tissue formation. Intergel (ferric hyaluronate) has been taken off the market for safety concerns
Baxter, Nottingham, UK	Icodextran 4%, Adept	There is insufficient evidence to recommend its use
Confluent Surgical, Waltham, MA, USA	Spraygel	There is insufficient evidence to recommend its use

Adapted from Ahmad G, Duffy JM, Farquhar C, et al. Barrier agents for adhesion prevention after gynaecological surgery. Cochrane Database Syst Rev 2008;(2):CD000475.

Table 2
Summary of barriers studied for the prevention of adhesions

Company	Product	Notes
Genzyme, Middleton, WI, USA	Seprafilm	Limited evidence in preventing adhesion following myomectomy
Johnson & Johnson, Somerville, NJ, USA	Interceed	Shown to reduce new and reformation of adhesions
W.L. Gore & Associates, Newark, DE, USA	GoreTex	Shown to be more effective than placebo and Interceed in the prevention of adhesions

Adapted from Farquhar C, Vandekerckhove P, Watson A, et al. Barrier agents for preventing adhesions after surgery for subfertility [systematic review]. Cochrane Database Syst Rev 2008;(2): CD000475.

surgery for being adhesiogenic,[68] but this has never been studied in comparison with ablation surgery for endometriosis. Good surgical technique is most important for minimizing adhesions, including achieving good hemostasis and minimizing char or desiccated tissue.[69] Adjunctives for adhesion prevention have been studied, and include the use of instillates[70] (**Table 1**) and barriers[71] (**Table 2**). Of all the barriers, GoreTex (W.L. Gore and Associates, Newark, DE, USA) has been shown to be the most effective, but it requires being secured in place and usually requires a second laparoscopy to remove it. There is some evidence to suggest that peritoneal closure may help to reduce adhesions in comparison with nonclosure.[72] Ovarian adhesions and ovarian surgery (such as cystectomy) are risk factors for developing new and recurrent adhesions.[68,73] In the General Surgery literature, Seprafilm (Genzyme, Middleton, WI, USA) has been shown to reduce abdominal adhesions,[74] and the use of a Seprafilm slurry has been described for its use at laparoscopy.[75] Further research is required to develop safe and effective adhesion prevention products.[76]

SUMMARY

Laparoscopic surgery has a clear, established role in the diagnosis and treatment of endometriosis of pelvic pain and infertility. Patients with pain (affecting quality of life), especially with infertility, should be offered diagnostic laparoscopy. A high index of suspicion will lead to early diagnosis and treatment of endometriosis, and better outcomes for patients. Excision surgery can more completely treat the disease than can ablation. Appropriate patient selection, and preoperative planning, will ideally lead to "see and treat" laparoscopy. The goal of laparoscopic management of endometriosis is the optimal removal or treatment of all visible lesions, both typical and atypical, and deep disease. Hysterectomy may be needed for suspicion of adenomyosis in patients with dysmenorrhea who have borne children, although ovarian conservation can be achieved if the endometriosis is optimally treated. Referral to a center or surgeon with expertise in the laparoscopic treatment of endometriosis is always an option for difficult cases or deep disease. The development of dedicated centers of expertise for treating endometriosis with appropriately trained surgeons and a committed multidisciplinary expert team is recommended.

SUPPLEMENTARY DATA

Video related to this article can be found online at http://dx.doi.org/10.1016/j.ogc.2014.05.002.

REFERENCES

1. Meuleman C, Vandenabeele B, Fieuws S, et al. High prevalence of endometriosis in infertile women with normal ovulation and normospermic partners. Fertil Steril 2009;92:68–74.
2. Rogers PA, D'Hooghe TM, Fazleabas A, et al. Priorities for endometriosis research: recommendations from an international consensus workshop. Reprod Sci 2009;16:335–46.
3. Nnoaham KE, Hummelshoj L, Webster P, et al. Impact of endometriosis on quality of life and work productivity: a multicenter study across ten countries. Fertil Steril 2011;96:366–73.e8.
4. Arruda MS, Petta CA, Abrao MS, et al. Time elapsed from onset of symptoms to diagnosis of endometriosis in a cohort study of Brazilian women. Hum Reprod 2003;18:756–9.
5. Hadfield R, Mardon H, Barlow D, et al. Delay in the diagnosis of endometriosis: a survey of women from the USA and the UK. Hum Reprod 1996;11: 878–80.
6. Ballard K, Lowton K, Wright J. What's the delay? A qualitative study of women's experiences of reaching a diagnosis of endometriosis. Fertil Steril 2006;86: 1296–301.
7. Janssen EB, Rijkers AC, Hoppenbrouwers K, et al. Prevalence of endometriosis diagnosed by laparoscopy in adolescents with dysmenorrhea or chronic pelvic pain: a systematic review. Hum Reprod Update 2013;19:570–82.
8. Brosens I, Gordts S, Benagiano G. Endometriosis in adolescents is a hidden, progressive and severe disease that deserves attention, not just compassion. Hum Reprod 2013;28(8):2026–31.
9. American College of Obstetricians and Gynecologists. ACOG Committee Opinion. Number 310, April 2005. Endometriosis in adolescents. Obstet Gynecol 2005;105(4):921–7.
10. Practice bulletin no. 114: management of endometriosis. Obstet Gynecol 2010; 116:223–36.
11. Yeung P Jr, Sinervo K, Winer W, et al. Complete laparoscopic excision of endometriosis in teenagers: is postoperative hormonal suppression necessary? Fertil Steril 2011;95(6):1909–12.
12. Yeung P Jr, Tu F, Bajzak K, et al. A pilot feasibility multicenter study of patients after excision of endometriosis. JSLS 2013;17:88–94.
13. Meuleman C, Tomassetti C, Gaspar Da Vitoria Magro M, et al. Laparoscopic treatment of endometriosis. Minerva Ginecol 2013;65:125–42.
14. Jarrell JF, Vilos GA, Allaire C, et al. Consensus guidelines for the management of chronic pelvic pain. J Obstet Gynaecol Can 2005;27:869–910.
15. American Fertility Society. Revised American Fertility Society classification of endometriosis. Fertil Steril 1985;43:351–2.
16. Vercellini P, Trespidi L, De Giorgi O, et al. Endometriosis and pelvic pain: relation to disease stage and localization. Fertil Steril 1996;65:299–304.
17. Fauconnier A, Chapron C, Dubuisson JB, et al. Relation between pain symptoms and the anatomic location of deep infiltrating endometriosis. Fertil Steril 2002;78:719–26.
18. Hsu AL, Sinaii N, Segars J, et al. Relating pelvic pain location to surgical findings of endometriosis. Obstet Gynecol 2011;118:223–30.
19. Adamson GD. Endometriosis classification: an update. Curr Opin Obstet Gynecol 2011;23:213–20.

20. Doyle JO, Missmer SA, Laufer MR. The effect of combined surgical-medical intervention on the progression of endometriosis in an adolescent and young adult population. J Pediatr Adolesc Gynecol 2009;22:257–63.
21. Chapron C, Souza C, Borghese B, et al. Oral contraceptives and endometriosis: the past use of oral contraceptives for treating severe primary dysmenorrhea is associated with endometriosis, especially deep infiltrating endometriosis. Hum Reprod 2011;26:2028–35.
22. Chapron C, Lafay-Pillet MC, Monceau E, et al. Questioning patients about their adolescent history can identify markers associated with deep infiltrating endometriosis. Fertil Steril 2011;95:877–81.
23. Chapron C, Borghese B, Streuli I, et al. Markers of adult endometriosis detectable in adolescence. J Pediatr Adolesc Gynecol 2011;24:S7–12.
24. Catenacci M, Sastry S, Falcone T. Laparoscopic surgery for endometriosis. Clin Obstet Gynecol 2009;52:351–61.
25. Practice Committee of the American Society for Reproductive Medicine. Endometriosis and infertility: a committee opinion. Fertil Steril 2012;98:591–8.
26. ACOG Committee on Practice Bulletins–Gynecology. ACOG Practice Bulletin No. 51. Chronic pelvic pain. Obstet Gynecol 2004;103:589–605.
27. Woolf CJ. Central sensitization: implications for the diagnosis and treatment of pain. Pain 2011;152:S2–15.
28. Practice Committee of the American Society for Reproductive Medicine. Endometriosis and infertility. Fertil Steril 2004;81:1441–6.
29. Johnson NP, Hummelshoj L, World Endometriosis Society Montpellier Consortium. Consensus on current management of endometriosis. Hum Reprod 2013;28(6): 1552–68.
30. Jacobson TZ, Barlow DH, Garry R, et al. Laparoscopic surgery for pelvic pain associated with endometriosis. Cochrane Database Syst Rev 2009;(4): CD001300.
31. Jacobson TZ, Barlow DH, Koninckx PR, et al. Laparoscopic surgery for subfertility associated with endometriosis. Cochrane Database Syst Rev 2010;(1): CD001398.
32. Lee HJ, Lee JE, Ku SY, et al. Natural conception rate following laparoscopic surgery in infertile women with endometriosis. Clin Exp Reprod Med 2013;40: 29–32.
33. Darai E, Marpeau O, Thomassin I, et al. Fertility after laparoscopic colorectal resection for endometriosis: preliminary results. Fertil Steril 2005;84:945–50.
34. Unger CA, Laufer MR. Progression of endometriosis in non-medically managed adolescents: a case series. J Pediatr Adolesc Gynecol 2011;24:e21–3.
35. Ball E, Koh C, Janik G, et al. Gynaecological laparoscopy: 'see and treat' should be the gold standard. Curr Opin Obstet Gynecol 2008;20:325–30.
36. Chapron C, Chopin N, Borghese B, et al. Surgical management of deeply infiltrating endometriosis: an update. Ann N Y Acad Sci 2004;1034:326–37.
37. Goncalves MO, Podgaec S, Dias JA Jr, et al. Transvaginal ultrasonography with bowel preparation is able to predict the number of lesions and rectosigmoid layers affected in cases of deep endometriosis, defining surgical strategy. Hum Reprod 2010;25:665–71.
38. Goncalves MO, Dias JA Jr, Podgaec S, et al. Transvaginal ultrasound for diagnosis of deeply infiltrating endometriosis. Int J Gynaecol Obstet 2009;104: 156–60.
39. Abrao MS, Podgaec S, Dias JA Jr, et al. Endometriosis lesions that compromise the rectum deeper than the inner muscularis layer have more than 40% of the

circumference of the rectum affected by the disease. J Minim Invasive Gynecol 2008;15:280–5.

40. Abrao MS, Goncalves MO, Dias JA Jr, et al. Comparison between clinical examination, transvaginal sonography and magnetic resonance imaging for the diagnosis of deep endometriosis. Hum Reprod 2007;22:3092–7.
41. Remorgida V, Ferrero S, Fulcheri E, et al. Bowel endometriosis: presentation, diagnosis, and treatment. Obstet Gynecol Surv 2007;62:461–70.
42. Redwine DB. Ovarian endometriosis: a marker for more extensive pelvic and intestinal disease. Fertil Steril 1999;72:310–5.
43. Minelli L, Ceccaroni M, Ruffo G, et al. Laparoscopic conservative surgery for stage IV symptomatic endometriosis: short-term surgical complications. Fertil Steril 2010;94:1218–22.
44. Albee RB Jr, Sinervo K, Fisher DT. Laparoscopic excision of lesions suggestive of endometriosis or otherwise atypical in appearance: relationship between visual findings and final histologic diagnosis. J Minim Invasive Gynecol 2008; 15:32–7.
45. Koninckx PR, Ussia A, Adamyan L, et al. Deep endometriosis: definition, diagnosis, and treatment. Fertil Steril 2012;98:564–71.
46. Hidaka T, Nakashima A, Hashimoto Y, et al. Effects of laparoscopic radical surgery for deep endometriosis on endometriosis-related pelvic pain. Minim Invasive Ther Allied Technol 2012;21:355–61.
47. Brouwer R, Woods RJ. Rectal endometriosis: results of radical excision and review of published work. ANZ J Surg 2007;77:562–71.
48. Vignali M, Bianchi S, Candiani M, et al. Surgical treatment of deep endometriosis and risk of recurrence. J Minim Invasive Gynecol 2005;12:508–13.
49. D'Hooghe T, Hummelshoj L. Multi-disciplinary centres/networks of excellence for endometriosis management and research: a proposal. Hum Reprod 2006; 21:2743–8.
50. Healey M, Ang WC, Cheng C. Surgical treatment of endometriosis: a prospective randomized double-blinded trial comparing excision and ablation. Fertil Steril 2010;94:2536–40.
51. Wright J, Lotfallah H, Jones K, et al. A randomized trial of excision versus ablation for mild endometriosis. Fertil Steril 2005;83:1830–6.
52. Garry R. The effectiveness of laparoscopic excision of endometriosis. Curr Opin Obstet Gynecol 2004;16:299–303.
53. Hart RJ, Hickey M, Maouris P, et al. Excisional surgery versus ablative surgery for ovarian endometriomata. Cochrane Database Syst Rev 2008;(2): CD004992.
54. Alborzi S, Ravanbakhsh R, Parsanezhad ME, et al. A comparison of follicular response of ovaries to ovulation induction after laparoscopic ovarian cystectomy or fenestration and coagulation versus normal ovaries in patients with endometrioma. Fertil Steril 2007;88:507–9.
55. Somigliana E, Berlanda N, Benaglia L, et al. Surgical excision of endometriomas and ovarian reserve: a systematic review on serum antimullerian hormone level modifications. Fertil Steril 2012;98:1531–8.
56. Raffi F, Metwally M, Amer S. The impact of excision of ovarian endometrioma on ovarian reserve: a systematic review and meta-analysis. J Clin Endocrinol Metab 2012;97:3146–54.
57. Litta P, D'Agostino G, Conte L, et al. Anti-Mullerian hormone trend after laparoscopic surgery in women with ovarian endometrioma. Gynecol Endocrinol 2013; 29:452–4.

58. Uncu G, Kasapoglu I, Ozerkan K, et al. Prospective assessment of the impact of endometriomas and their removal on ovarian reserve and determinants of the rate of decline in ovarian reserve. Hum Reprod 2013;28(8):2140–5.
59. Raffi F, Shaw RW, Amer SA. National survey of the current management of endometriomas in women undergoing assisted reproductive treatment. Hum Reprod 2012;27:2712–9.
60. Eskicioglu C, Forbes SS, Fenech DS, et al. Preoperative bowel preparation for patients undergoing elective colorectal surgery: a clinical practice guideline endorsed by the Canadian Society of Colon and Rectal Surgeons. Can J Surg 2010;53:385–95.
61. Guenaga KF, Matos D, Wille-Jorgensen P. Mechanical bowel preparation for elective colorectal surgery. Cochrane Database Syst Rev 2011;(9):CD001544.
62. Morelli M, Venturella R, Zullo F. Risk-reducing salpingectomy as a new and safe strategy to prevent ovarian cancer. Am J Obstet Gynecol 2013;209:395–6.
63. Sutton CJ, Ewen SP, Whitelaw N, et al. Prospective, randomized, double-blind, controlled trial of laser laparoscopy in the treatment of pelvic pain associated with minimal, mild, and moderate endometriosis [see comment]. Fertil Steril 1994;62:696–700.
64. Winkel CA. Evaluation and management of women with endometriosis. Obstet Gynecol 2003;102:397–408.
65. Guo SW. Recurrence of endometriosis and its control. Hum Reprod Update 2009;15:441–61.
66. Schnuriger B, Barmparas G, Branco BC, et al. Prevention of postoperative peritoneal adhesions: a review of the literature. Am J Surg 2011;201:111–21.
67. Alpay Z, Saed GM, Diamond MP. Postoperative adhesions: from formation to prevention. Semin Reprod Med 2008;26:313–21.
68. Parker JD, Sinaii N, Segars JH, et al. Adhesion formation after laparoscopic excision of endometriosis and lysis of adhesions. Fertil Steril 2005;84:1457–61.
69. Practice Committee of American Society for Reproductive Medicine in collaboration with Society of Reproductive Surgeons. Pathogenesis, consequences, and control of peritoneal adhesions in gynecologic surgery: a committee opinion. Fertil Steril 2013;99:1550–5.
70. Metwally M, Watson A, Lilford R, et al. Fluid and pharmacological agents for adhesion prevention after gynaecological surgery [systematic review]. Cochrane Database Syst Rev 2007;(2):CD001298.
71. Ahmad G, Duffy JM, Farquhar C, et al. Barrier agents for adhesion prevention after gynaecological surgery. Cochrane Database Syst Rev 2008;(2): CD000475.
72. Cheong YC, Premkumar G, Metwally M, et al. To close or not to close? A systematic review and a meta-analysis of peritoneal non-closure and adhesion formation after caesarean section. Eur J Obstet Gynecol Reprod Biol 2009;147:3–8.
73. De Wilde RL, Brolmann H, Koninckx PR, et al. Prevention of adhesions in gynaecological surgery: the 2012 European field guideline. Gynecol Surg 2012;9:365–8.
74. Zeng Q, Yu Z, You J, et al. Efficacy and safety of Seprafilm for preventing postoperative abdominal adhesion: systematic review and meta-analysis. World J Surg 2007;31:2125–31 [discussion: 32].
75. Ortiz MV, Awad ZT. An easy technique for laparoscopic placement of Seprafilm. Surg Laparosc Endosc Percutan Tech 2009;19:e181–3.
76. Diamond MP, Wexner SD, diZereg GS, et al. Adhesion prevention and reduction: current status and future recommendations of a multinational interdisciplinary consensus conference. Surg Innov 2010;17:183–8.

Interstitial Cystitis

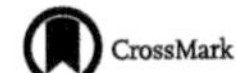

Epidemiology, Pathophysiology, and Clinical Presentation

Mary T. McLennan, MD

KEYWORDS

- Interstitial cystitis • Painful bladder syndrome
- Chronic pelvic pain • Urgency/frequency • Nocturia

KEY POINTS

- Interstitial cystitis is commonly underdiagnosed.
- Patients with lower abdominal/pelvic pain or discomfort should be specifically questioned about associated symptoms such as frequency, urgency, and nocturia.
- Nocturia in a young patient is abnormal, and this should lead the clinician to rule out interstitial cystitis as a possible cause for the pain.
- Dyspareunia is also common in these patients.
- There is a high association with other chronic pain conditions.
- The etiology is still unknown, although there may be a bladder mucosal defect plus either central sensitization of the spinal cord or a sensory processing disorder.

INTRODUCTION

It is difficult to discuss a particular disorder when there is no universally accepted name or definition of the disorder. Interstitial cystitis (IC) is recognized by providers as a chronic painful bladder condition; however, it has several synonyms depending on where in the world the physician practices and which organization defines the entity.

The National Institute of Diabetes and Digestive and Kidney Diseases defined IC by strict criteria to ensure that consistent patient populations were studied, being intended for research. The patient must have glomerulations or classic Hunner ulcers on cystoscopic examination, and pain associated with either bladder filling or urinary urgency. There must be at least 10 glomerulations per quadrant in at least 3 quadrants after distention of the bladder was under anesthesia to 80 to 100 cm of water pressure for 1 to 2 minutes. Presence of any of the criteria in **Box 1** excludes the diagnosis of

The author has nothing to disclose.
Obstetrics Gynecology and Women's Health, Saint Louis University School of Medicine, 6420 Clayton Road, St Louis, MO 63117, USA
E-mail address: mclennan@slu.edu

Obstet Gynecol Clin N Am 41 (2014) 385–395
http://dx.doi.org/10.1016/j.ogc.2014.05.004 **obgyn.theclinics.com**
0889-8545/14/$ – see front matter

Box 1
National Institutes of Health exclusion criteria

1. Bladder capacity greater than 350 mL on awake cystometry using either a gas or liquid filling medium
2. Absence of an intense urge to void with the bladder filled to 100 mL gas or 150 mL water during cystometry, using a fill rate of 30 to 100 mL per minute
3. The demonstration of phasic involuntary bladder contractions on cystometry using the fill rate described previously
4. Duration of symptoms less than 9 months
5. Absence of nocturia
6. Symptoms relieved by antimicrobials, urinary antiseptics, anticholinergics, or antispasmodics
7. A frequency of urination, while awake, of less than 8 times a day
8. A diagnosis of bacterial cystitis or prostatitis within a 3-month period
9. Bladder or ureteral calculi
10. Active genital herpes
11. Uterine, cervical, vaginal, or urethral cancer
12. Urethral diverticulum
13. Cyclophosphamide or any type of chemical cystitis
14. Tuberculous cystitis
15. Radiation cystitis
16. Benign or malignant bladder tumors
17. Vaginitis
18. Age less than 18 years

IC.[1] Unfortunately, because of the diversity of symptoms it is apparent that such exclusion criteria would exclude a large number of patients who likely have IC. Hanno and colleagues[2] reported that applying these strict criteria missed diagnosing more than 60% of patients regarded by experienced clinicians as definitely or likely having IC.

The American Urological Association (AUA) released its evidence-based guidelines for IC/bladder pain syndrome (BPS) in the hopes of improving early diagnosis and treatment. IC/BPS (both used) was defined as an "unpleasant sensation (pain, pressure), perceived to be related to the urinary bladder, associated with lower urinary tract symptoms of more than 6 weeks duration in the absence of infection or other identifiable causes."[3] One can see from this definition that symptom duration is very short, and this interpretation was deliberately selected to allow for treatment after a relatively short period of symptoms. The Society for Urodynamics and Female Urology concurred, stating that their definition constituted a clinical strategy and was not intended to be interpreted rigidly.[4]

The International Society for the Study of Bladder Pain Syndrome defines the disorder as chronic pelvic pain, pressure, or discomfort perceived to be related to the urinary bladder, accompanied by at least one other urinary symptom such as persistent urge to void or urinary frequency. Confusable diseases as a cause of symptoms must be excluded by history, physical examination, urinalysis, urine cultures, uroflowmetry, postvoid residual, cystoscopy, and biopsy if indicated.[5]

The European Association of Urology (EAU) embraces the term BPS, recommending the term IC be reserved for a subset of patients with verified signs of chronic inflammation extending submucosally, based at the time of cystoscopy, hydrodistention, and bladder biopsy. It recommends that BPS is diagnosed on the bases of symptoms, examination, urinalysis, and cystoscopy, with hydrodistention and biopsy. Pain should be persistent or recurrent over a 6-month period to be defined as chronic. The character of the pain is key to the diagnosis, with pain typically related to bladder filling, increasing with increased bladder volume, typically located suprapubically, but sometimes radiating to the groin, vagina, rectum, and sacrum. Pain is relieved by voiding but returns shortly with further bladder filling. The EAU recognizes that the character of the pain is key to the symptoms, and that patients typically have frequency and always have nocturia. Although nocturia is a consistent symptom across age groups, its incidence does vary with age, thus making this definition potentially exclusive to a certain subgroup of patients (see later discussion of clinical presentation).[6]

A consensus panel in Asia defined IC as a disease of the urinary bladder, diagnosed by 3 conditions: "lower urinary tract symptoms, bladder pathology, and exclusion of confusable diseases." The characteristic symptom of this complex is termed hypersensitive bladder syndrome (HBS), which is defined as "bladder hypersensitivity usually associated with urinary frequency with or without bladder pain." Included in this was an algorithm for diagnosis and management of this condition.[7]

Irrespective of the definition the clinician adopts, there appear to be certain consistencies across them: unpleasant sensation or chronic pain, and pressure or discomfort that is perceived to be related to the bladder accompanied by some other urinary symptom, most notably urge to void, frequency, or nocturia. The biggest difference in definition appears to be the time required to establish the diagnosis, which ranges from 6 weeks for the AUA to "chronic" for the EAU (6 months). Cystoscopy is included in most criteria to allow classification and further management strategies; however, the AUA differs in that cystoscopy is listed as a consideration and not a requirement. The AUA guidelines do not rely on the presence or absence of glomerulations; however, the presence of Hunner ulcers allows directed treatment.

PREVALENCE

Prevalence data are difficult to obtain because they depend on the definition, the population studied, and the method. Prevalence appears to have changed significantly over the past 40 years or so. In a population-based study in 1975 the reported prevalence was 10 per 100,000 (0.01%), compared with 30 per 100,000 in (0.03%) in 1987 and 510 per 100,000 (0.5%) in 1994.[8] In a cross-sectional study of the Boston area from 2002 to 2005, the prevalence of painful bladder syndrome was 2.6%. The definition was based on self-report of pain which increased with bladder filling and was relieved by urination present for at least 3 months.[9] In 2011 Berry and colleagues[10] published a study using 2006 United States census data. The random sample included 131,691 adult females. Of these, 32,474 women reported having bladder symptoms or diagnoses, of whom 12,752 completed the questionnaires. Depending on the definition used, the prevalence ranged from 2.7% for a high-specificity definition (83% for distinguishing cases that did not have bladder pain syndrome from those with other bladder and pelvic pain) to 6.5% for a high-sensitivity definition (81% chance for identifying cases diagnosed with bladder pain syndrome). These percentages translate into 3.3 to 7.9 million United States women 18 years or older with BPS/IC symptoms.[10] Only 9.7% of these patients reported being given a diagnosis of BPS/IC, underscoring the potential for underdiagnosis.

ETIOLOGY

Urothelial and Epithelial Dysfunction

In patients undergoing cystoscopy for potential IC, epithelial abnormalities can be seen in the form of glomerulations and/or Hunner ulcers. The bladder urothelium is lined by a protective layer of dense glycosaminoglycans (GAG), which maintains impermeability to various solutes in the urine. The basic characteristic of this layer is to provide mechanical and electrostatic defense against penetration by toxic, acidic, or infective agents. This property is thought to be the basis of why the instillation of potassium (K sensitivity test) into the bladder of patients with IC will increase or mimic the symptoms in most patients, an attribute that can also be seen in patients with mucosal defects from radiation cystitis.[11–14] However, studies have failed to demonstrate any difference in the total GAG levels between controls and those with IC.[14,15] However, most GAG found in the urine appears to be produced in the upper tract, so it is uncertain as to whether a difference would be expected to be found.

Tamm-Horsfall Protein

Tamm-Horsfall protein (THP) is an anionic protein that binds and neutralizes urinary toxins, providing a protective function in the bladder. It is hypothesized that abnormal THP proteins may play a role in the pathogenesis of IC. It has been demonstrated that compared with normal subjects those with THP protein have reduced sialic acid content, which is critical to its protective activity.[15,16] This deficiency may affect the neutralization of toxic factors in the urine. There is additional evidence that the levels of urinary cationic metabolites are higher in patients with IC and potentially cause more damage to the bladder wall, resulting in a double insult.

Heparin and pentosan polysulfate have both been shown to neutralize toxic factors, and this may help to explain their effect as going beyond simply that on the GAG layer as initially thought.[15,16]

Mast Cell Activation

Biopsies of the bladder wall have demonstrated increased numbers and activation of mast cells. These cells contain inflammatory mediators such as histamine, leukotrienes, serotonins, and cytokines.[14,17] Mast cells are thought to potentially play a role in frequency, pain, and fibrosis, and forms the basis for the use of antihistamines for the treatment of IC.

Infection

Patients will often relate a history of having an acute urinary tract infection that initiated pain, and that symptoms failed to resolve with antibiotics. However, culture-proven urinary tract infections are found in the minority of patients.[18,19] The potential sensitization of the bladder arising from the inflammation caused by a urinary tract infection may be contributory, but its role remains unknown.

Antiproliferative Factor

Bladder epithelial cells of IC patients produce a novel antiproliferative factor (APF). The normal bladder epithelium does not produce this factor in vitro. APF can inhibit the proliferation of normal bladder epithelial cells, making it a possible cause of epithelial thinning. It may alter the differentiation of tight junction formation and proliferation of bladder epithelial cells, resulting in a decreased epithelial barrier. Moreover, APF decreases heparin-binding epidermal growth factor, which is important in the initiation of cell migration for epithelial repair.[20]

Genetics

It has been reported in twin studies that there is a higher concordance of IC among monozygotic than dizygotic twins. In addition, adult first-degree relatives of a patient with painful bladder syndrome have a 17 times higher rate of IC than the general population.[21]

Autoimmunity

The role of autoimmune deficiency has not been determined. However, $CD8^+$ and $CD4^+$ lymphocytes, B lymphocytes, plasma cells, and immunoglobulins (IgA, IgG, and IgM) have been found to be more prevalent in the bladder wall of IC patients than in controls.[22–24]

Central Sensitization of the Spinal Cord

Because of the increased incidence of other chronic pelvic pain syndromes along with IC, it has been theorized that all of these disorders may represent central sensitization of the lower spinal cord. This proposition suggests that non–bladder-related syndromes that cause pelvic pain would initiate sensitization in the lower spinal cord such that the bladder was also perceived as a site of pain. This central sensitization leads to upregulation in the dorsal horn such that the noxious stimulus may subsequently be removed while the pain is still perceived from the organ/origin. Upregulation may also lead to a decreased threshold for activation, leading to perception of pain at lower levels of stimulation. This inference might help to explain why patients with IC have significant discomfort with very small bladder volumes in comparison with normal subjects, and why patients still have pain after cystectomy. It also lends validity to the use of neuropathic agents in the treatment of IC, especially those that do not affect the bladder per se. However, it does not explain the association with extrapelvic nonbladder pain syndromes such as chronic fatigue and fibromyalgia.[21,25]

Sensory Processing

As noted earlier, the close association with other chronic pain syndromes unrelated to the pelvis is not adequately explained by a local bladder disorder or central sensitization. An alternative hypothesis is that these patients have abnormal sensory processing. It has been demonstrated that in patients undergoing thoracic surgery, those with preexisting abnormal sensory processing continue to have chronic postoperative pain. By contrast, patients having a hip replacement for hip osteoarthritis noted hyperanalgesia in other sites normalized after replacement.[25–27] Warren and colleagues[25] have published an interesting article on the possible etiology and pathophysiologic processes in nonbladder pain syndromes and IC.

CLINICAL PRESENTATION

Early teachings were that this was a disease of young, reproductive-age women. However, recent studies in multiple different countries have shown that it occurs across all ages. In a diverse population in Denmark, the age at diagnosis ranged from 16 to 88 years, with a median age of 53 years.[28] In a recent cohort of 3397 community-dwelling women who met the RAND IC epidemiology case definition, age ranged from 18 to 92 years, with a mean age of 45.7 years for a high-sensitivity case definition and 46.4 years for a high-specificity definition.[29]

Symptoms tend to vary across age distributions. For those younger than 30 years daytime frequency is the most common presenting symptom, followed equally by dysuria and urgency. For those 30 to 50 years old, nocturia is most predominant followed by daytime frequency and dysuria, with dyspareunia and vulvar pain far less frequent at approximately 20% lower rates than for the younger age group. For those 60 years or older, nocturia is the most frequent symptom. Dyspareunia and vulvar pain occur with less frequency than either of the 2 younger groups (**Table 1**).[30]

In terms of key indicators for the practicing physician, nocturia in a young patient with pelvic pain should raise the index of suspicion for IC. Rates range from 50% to 70%.[28,30] It is also important that dyspareunia is reported in up to 60% of young patients.[30] Pain is not specifically related to intercourse, with 40% complaining of bladder pain after intercourse and an equal number reporting exacerbation of bladder symptoms. Approximately one-third of patients may have pain located anywhere within the genital area. In a study of 1469 patients who completed bladder-specific and general sexual dysfunction questionnaires, Bogart and colleagues[27] noted that the majority (88%) with a current partner endorsed 1 or more symptom of general sexual dysfunction in the previous 4 weeks. Bladder pain during and/or after sex was the most prevalent symptom; however, 65% of patients reported lack of sexual interest. This percentage is approximately double that of the general United States population.[31] Only one-fourth of these women had sought any medical help for this sexual dysfunction.

The classic description is pain that increases with increasing bladder volume and is relieved temporarily by voiding. Warren and colleagues[32] noted that 75% of patients reported that pain was worse with filling; however, an additional 9% noted that their pain improved with bladder filling. Two-thirds of reported pain was suprapubic (83%), urethral (36%), genital (23%), and nongenital (23%).[26]

Urinary frequency is another consistent symptom across the various age groups, with one study reporting 86% of patients having frequency greater than 11 times during a 24-hour period and 71% having nocturia 3 or more times at night.[32] Other investigators reported nocturia occurring at least 4 times in 15% and 44% of cases.[28]

Up to 90% of patients report that certain foods and drinks may aggravate or flare their IC. Friedlander and colleagues[33] reported that questionnaire-based literature suggests that citrus fruits, tomatoes, vitamin C, artificial sweeteners, coffee, tea, carbonated alcoholic beverages, and spicy foods tend to exacerbate symptoms, whereas sodium bicarbonate and calcium glycerophosphate (Prelief) tend to improve symptoms. Chocolate, coffee, and tea have also been noted to be problematic for some patients, although the exact mechanism is uncertain. Alcohol also seems to be a trigger, and in one study 94% of patients reported worsening of symptoms after drinking an alcoholic beverage.[33] White wine seems to be better than red, light beer better than dark, and whiskey and brandy better than tequila and vodka. Lists of foods can be found on various Web sites. As there is such a variability between patients, the

Table 1
Variation with age

	<30 y	30–59 y	>60 y
Urgency	73	56	52
Frequency	79	55	58
Dysuria	73	42	52
Nocturia	49	64	76
Dyspareunia	62	30	23
Vulvar pain	47	27	21

Data from Hanno PM, Landis JR, Matthews-Cook Y, et al. The diagnosis of interstitial cystitis revisited: lessons learned from the National Institutes of Health Interstitial Cystitis Database study. J Urol 1999;161(2):553–7.

author would typically recommend that if the patient ingests a particular food or beverage on the "bad list" they should desist for 1 week, see if it makes any difference to their symptoms, and if not add it back and sequentially delete another. The alternative is to cut everything out and then gradually add them back a week at a time; however, this is often very prohibitive for patients, as the list is so inclusive and compliance poorer than when asking them to eliminate one item at a time.

ASSOCIATION WITH NONBLADDER PAIN SYNDROMES

There have been numerous and consistent reports on the association of IC with other chronic pain conditions. However, it is difficult to discern the antecedent disorder that may point to a common etiology or trigger.

Fibromyalgia

It has been reported that 9% to 12% of patients with IC also experience fibromyalgia, and that 2.25% to 27% of patients with fibromyalgia have symptoms consistent with IC.[34] Nickel and colleagues[24] noted in a case-control study a high association between IC and fibromyalgia at approximately 18% versus 70.7%. In a recent question-based screening for 4 different pain conditions in the Michigan Women's Health study, the odds of having fibromyalgia with a diagnosis of IC was 5.1 (95% confidence interval [CI] 3.2–8.1).[35] In a case-control study of 313 patients with urologic symptoms/signs and characteristics of IC compared with matched controls, fibromyalgia, chronic fatigue syndrome, irritable bowel syndrome, and Sicca syndrome were consistently associated with one another. Seventy-eight percent of the patients with IC had more than 2 syndromes, compared with 45% of the control group. The investigators concluded that there were 3 possible explanations: (1) there was no direct relationship but there was sharing of a genetic or environmental risk factor; (2) based on the antecedent syndrome itself, the other syndromes were a risk factor for development of IC; and (3) the particular syndrome and IC were different manifestations of the same pathophysiology or disease.[36]

Chronic Fatigue

In the study of twin discordant pairs for various definitions of chronic fatigue, the fatigued twin was 20 times more likely to have IC than the nonfatigued twin.[34] Nickel and colleagues[24] reported chronic fatigue in 9.5% of those with IC versus 1.7% in controls matched for age. Warren and colleagues[37] also noted that antecedent nonbladder syndromes appear to be a risk factor for IC. The odds ratio of IC with chronic fatigue syndrome was 2.5, which was similar to that of all the chronic pain syndromes (2 and 2.9). The odds ratio of IC also increased with an increasing number of antecedent nonbladder pain syndromes.

Irritable Bowel

In one study of those with vulvodynia and other chronic comorbid pain conditions, those with irritable bowel had an odds ratio of 6.1 (95% CI 4.0–9.4) of having IC.[35] In a comparative study of the prevalence of nonbladder syndromes in IC patients versus matched controls, the odds ratio of irritable bowel based on self-reported physician diagnosis was 3.6 (95% CI 2.3–5.6) and 2.9 (95% CI 1.9–4.5) based on symptoms.[36] In a review of 1037 full-length published articles from 1966 to April 2008, Rodriguez and colleagues[34] reported that depending on the methodology used, between 7% and 48% of patients with IC or symptoms of BPS had irritable bowel, and patients with IC were 11 times more likely than controls to be diagnosed with irritable bowel. The most robust evidence for overlapping conditions existed between these 2 particular conditions, and the results were consistent across numerous studies and publications.

Other Gynecologic Pain Conditions

There has been an increase in reported association of other gynecologic syndromes with IC. A recent publication from a large vulvar center noted that the odds of screening positive for vulvodynia increased 2.3- to 3.3-fold when women reported having any of the 3 other chronic pain conditions (IC, irritable bowel, fibromyalgia). Patients with vulvodynia were also more likely to have IC or irritable bowel as their sole comorbidity.[26] However, it is difficult to discern whether this represents true vulvodynia or if it is referred pain of bladder origin.

Warren and colleagues[36] reported that after the onset of IC, 27% of their patients reported burning genital pain that worsened with touch, tampons, and coitus, which is consistent with vulvodynia; however, they considered this was best explained as referred pain. No explanation as to why the investigators believed it was "referred" was given.

In an interesting study during which patients were asked to map their pain on a whole-body diagram, IC patients reported greater frequency of pain in almost all body areas in comparison with controls. Twenty-seven percent of patients reported pain in what was described as the primary IC site (vagina, lower abdomen, lower back, pelvis, and buttock) while 23% reported primary pain site plus pain in 1 to 3 additional locations, 24% in 4 to 9 additional locations, and 26% in greater than 10 additional locations. In addition, they reported more severe sensory pain than the controls, and this increased further when pain was reported in more than 3 locations. IC patients also had higher scores on catastrophizing and depression. The investigators opined that as 73% of patients reported pain at an area outside of the primary IC, this indicated there may be some centrally mediated mechanism for the pain.[38]

In a 10-year review of the gynecologic literature assessing the prevalence of bladder pain and endometriosis,[39] the term "evil twin syndrome" was coined. The coexistence of IC and endometriosis ranged from 16% to 78% (average 48%). These investigators concluded that physicians who deal with patients with chronic pelvic pain need to investigate for IC in patients with endometriosis.

In a study of an existing database of patients with IC, Warren and colleagues[40] noted that in the 1 month before the diagnosis of IC, 38.7% of patients had a high incidence of hysterectomy, oophorectomy, and other pelvic surgeries. The approximate annual incidence of nonbladder pelvic surgeries was 15 times higher and that of hysterectomy 25 times higher than the incidence of the previous year, and higher than that of controls. This high rate of surgery declined over the first 2 years after diagnosis. Once the patient had a diagnosis of IC, surgery rates were markedly less, returning to the levels of those of controls over 2 years. Although this is only one report, those of us in clinical practice consistently hear from patients that they have had gynecologic surgeries, notably hysterectomy or oophorectomy, for their pelvic pain and that their pain was not relieved. This fact underscores the need for heightened awareness that there are other causes of pelvic pain other than the reproductive organs. Treating for IC or performing cystoscopy and hydrodistention are very low-level morbidity options compared with major gynecologic surgery.[41]

SUMMARY

For the practicing clinician, the important message is to consider IC/BPS in any patient with persistent pelvic or lower abdominal discomfort, particularly in the setting of any bladder symptom. This article underscores the importance of asking specifically about pain with bladder filling, urgency, frequency, and nocturia, and placing this diagnosis on the differential diagnosis of chronic pelvic pain. As there appears to be a high association with other chronic pain syndromes, it is useful to ask about any history of fibromyalgia, chronic fatigue, irritable bowel syndrome, endometriosis, and vulvodynia.

REFERENCES

1. Gillenwater JY, Wein AJ. Summary of the National Institute of Arthritis, Diabetes, Digestive and Kidney Diseases Workshop on Interstitial Cystitis, National Institutes of Health, Bethesda, Maryland, August 28-29, 1987. J Urol 1988;140(1):203–6.
2. Hanno PM, Landis JR, Matthews-Cook Y, et al. The diagnosis of interstitial cystitis revisited: lessons learned from the National Institutes of Health Interstitial Cystitis Database study. J Urol 1999;161(2):553–7.
3. Hanno PM, Burks DA, Clemens JQ, et al, Interstitial Cystitis Guidelines Panel of the American Urological Association Education and Research, Inc. AUA guideline for the diagnosis and treatment of interstitial cystitis/bladder pain syndrome. J Urol 2011;185(6):2162–70.
4. Hanno P, Andersson KE, Birder L, et al. Chronic pelvic pain syndrome/bladder pain syndrome: taking stock, looking ahead: ICI-RS 2011. Neurourol Urodyn 2012;31(3):375–83.
5. van de Merwe JP, Nordling J, Bouchelouche P, et al. Diagnostic criteria, classification, and nomenclature for painful bladder syndrome/interstitial cystitis: an ESSIC proposal. Eur Urol 2008;53(1):60–7.
6. Fall M, Baranowski AP, Elneil S, et al, European Association of Urology. EAU guidelines on chronic pelvic pain. Eur Urol 2010;57(1):35–48.
7. Homma Y, Ueda T, Tomoe H, et al, Interstitial cystitis guideline committee. Clinical guidelines for interstitial cystitis and hypersensitive bladder syndrome. Int J Urol 2009;16(7):597–615.
8. Jones CA, Nyberg L. Epidemiology of interstitial cystitis. Urology 1997;49(Suppl 5A): 2–9.
9. Hall SA, Link CL, Pulliam SJ, et al. The relationship of common medical conditions and medication use with symptoms of painful bladder syndrome: results from the Boston area community health survey. J Urol 2008;180(2):593–8.
10. Berry SH, Elliott MN, Suttorp M, et al. Prevalence of symptoms of bladder pain syndrome/interstitial cystitis among adult females in the United States. J Urol 2011;186(2):540–4.
11. Hurst RE. Structure, function, and pathology of proteoglycans and glycosaminoglycans in the urinary tract. World J Urol 1994;12(1):3–10.
12. Parsons CL, Stein PC, Bidair M, et al. Abnormal sensitivity to intravesical potassium in interstitial cystitis and radiation cystitis. Neurourol Urodyn 1994;13(5): 515–20.
13. Parsons CL, Lilly JD, Stein P. Epithelial dysfunction in nonbacterial cystitis (interstitial cystitis). J Urol 1991;145(4):732–5.
14. Vij M, Srikrishna S, Cardozo L. Interstitial cystitis: diagnosis and management. Eur J Obstet Gynecol Reprod Biol 2012;161(1):1–7.
15. Parsons CL, Shaw T, Berecz Z, et al. Role of urinary cations in the etiology of bladder symptoms and interstitial cystitis. BJU Int 2013. http://dx.doi.org/10.1111/bju.12603.
16. Argade S, Shaw T, Su Y, et al. Tamm-Horsfall protein-associated nucleotides in patients with interstitial cystitis. BJU Int 2013;111(5):811–9.

17. Peeker R, Enerbäck L, Fall M, et al. Recruitment, distribution and phenotypes of mast cells in interstitial cystitis. J Urol 2000;163(3):1009–15.
18. Warren JW, Brown V, Jacobs S, et al. Urinary tract infection and inflammation at onset of interstitial cystitis/painful bladder syndrome. Urology 2008;71(6): 1085–90.
19. Potts JM, Ward AM, Rackley RR. Association of chronic urinary symptoms in women and Ureaplasma urealyticum. Urology 2000;55(4):486–9.
20. Keay S. Cell signaling in interstitial cystitis/painful bladder syndrome. Cell Signal 2008;20(12):2174–9.
21. Warren JW, Jackson TL, Langenberg P, et al. Prevalence of interstitial cystitis in first-degree relatives of patients with interstitial cystitis. Urology 2004;63(1): 17–21.
22. MacDermott JP, Miller CH, Levy N, et al. Cellular immunity in interstitial cystitis. J Urol 1991;145(2):274–8.
23. Liebert M, Wedemeyer G, Stein JA, et al. Evidence for urothelial cell activation in interstitial cystitis. J Urol 1993;149(3):470–5.
24. Nickel JC, Tripp DA, Pontari M, et al. Interstitial cystitis/painful bladder syndrome and associated medical conditions with an emphasis on irritable bowel syndrome, fibromyalgia and chronic fatigue syndrome. J Urol 2010;184(4):1358–63.
25. Warren JW, van de Merwe JP, Nickel JC. Interstitial cystitis/bladder pain syndrome and nonbladder syndromes: facts and hypotheses. Urology 2011;78(4): 727–32.
26. Yarnitsky D, Crispel Y, Eisenberg E, et al. Prediction of chronic post-operative pain: pre-operative DNIC testing identifies patients at risk. Pain 2008;138(1): 22–8.
27. Bogart LM, Suttorp MJ, Elliott MN, et al. Prevalence and correlates of sexual dysfunction among women with bladder pain syndrome/interstitial cystitis. Urology 2011;77(3):576–80.
28. Richter B, Hesse U, Hansen AB, et al. Bladder pain syndrome/interstitial cystitis in a Danish population: a study using the 2008 criteria of the European Society for the Study of Interstitial Cystitis. BJU Int 2010;105(5):660–7.
29. Konkle KS, Berry SH, Elliott MN, et al. Comparison of an interstitial cystitis/ bladder pain syndrome clinical cohort with symptomatic community women from the RAND Interstitial Cystitis Epidemiology study. J Urol 2012;187(2): 508–12.
30. Rais-Bahrami S, Friedlander JI, Herati AS, et al. Symptom profile variability of interstitial cystitis/painful bladder syndrome by age. BJU Int 2012;109(9): 1356–9.
31. Laumann EO, Paik A, Rosen RC. Sexual dysfunction in the United States: prevalence and predictors. JAMA 1999;281(6):537–44.
32. Warren JW, Meyer WA, Greenberg P, et al. Using the International Continence Society's definition of painful bladder syndrome. Urology 2006;67(6):1138–42.
33. Friedlander JI, Shorter B, Moldwin RM. Diet and its role in interstitial cystitis/ bladder pain syndrome (IC/BPS) and comorbid conditions. BJU Int 2012; 109(11):1584–91.
34. Rodríguez MA, Afari N, Buchwald DS, National Institute of Diabetes and Digestive and Kidney Diseases Working Group on Urological Chronic Pelvic Pain. Evidence for overlap between urological and nonurological unexplained clinical conditions. J Urol 2009;182(5):2123–31.
35. Reed BD, Harlow SD, Sen A, et al. Relationship between vulvodynia and chronic comorbid pain conditions. Obstet Gynecol 2012;120(1):145–51.

36. Warren JW, Howard FM, Cross RK, et al. Antecedent nonbladder syndromes in case-control study of interstitial cystitis/painful bladder syndrome. Urology 2009;73(1):52–7.
37. Warren JW, Wesselmann U, Morozov V, et al. Numbers and types of nonbladder syndromes as risk factors for interstitial cystitis/painful bladder syndrome. Urology 2011;77(2):313–9.
38. Tripp DA, Nickel JC, Wong J, et al. Mapping of pain phenotypes in female patients with bladder pain syndrome/interstitial cystitis and controls. Eur Urol 2012;62(6):1188–94.
39. Tirlapur SA, Kuhrt K, Chaliha C, et al. The 'evil twin syndrome' in chronic pelvic pain: a systematic review of prevalence studies of bladder pain syndrome and endometriosis. Int J Surg 2013;11(3):233–7.
40. Warren JW, Howard FM, Morozov VV. Is there a high incidence of hysterectomy and other nonbladder surgeries before and after onset of interstitial cystitis/bladder pain syndrome? Am J Obstet Gynecol 2013;208(1):77.
41. Ingber MS, Peters KM, Killinger KA, et al. Dilemmas in diagnosing pelvic pain: multiple pelvic surgeries common in women with interstitial cystitis. Int Urogynecol J Pelvic Floor Dysfunct 2008;19(3):341–5.

Diagnosis and Management of Interstitial Cystitis

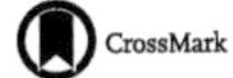

Susan Barr, MD

KEYWORDS

- Interstitial cystitis • Painful bladder syndrome • Bladder pain • Diagnosis of IC • Treatment of IC

KEY POINTS

- Interstitial cystitis is a diagnosis of exclusion.
- Cystoscopy and hydrodistension can provide additional therapeutic benefit in addition to being diagnostic.
- Adding bladder training at the time of cystoscopy and hydrodistension may help prolong the therapeutic benefit.
- Treatment options include oral therapy, intravesical therapy, and surgical approaches.
- Re-evaluating with objective measure, such as validated questionnaire, is important in deciding when a treatment regimen is not working.
- Using a multidisciplinary approach is optimal.

DIAGNOSIS

Patient History

History is key to considering a potential diagnosis. As noted in the article in this issue by McLennan, symptoms may vary with age, but the typical patient with interstitial cystitis (IC) has urinary frequency, urgency, nocturia, and bladder or pelvic pain or pressure. The patient may start with only one of these symptoms and advance over time. Patients sometimes will describe a "peeing glass" sensation with voiding but also have improvement in pain after voiding. IC/painful bladder syndrome (PBS) is also a potential cause of sexual pain and should be on the differential when a patient presents with the complaint of dyspareunia. Thirty-five percent of the IC patients reported an effect on their sexual life.[1] Patients will typically describe dietary triggers. "Pain that worsened with certain food or drink and/or worsened with bladder filling and/or improved with urination" was described by 97% of IC/PBS patients.[2]

Pain often distinguishes IC from overactive bladder. Vulvar pain should differentiate vulvodynia from IC. Dysmenorrhea distinguishes endometriosis from IC.

The author has nothing to disclose.

Division of Urogynecology, Department of Obstetrics and Gynecology, University of Arkansas for Medical Sciences, 4301 West Markham, Slot 518, Little Rock, AR 72205, USA
E-mail address: SABarr@uams.edu

Obstet Gynecol Clin N Am 41 (2014) 397–407
http://dx.doi.org/10.1016/j.ogc.2014.04.001 **obgyn.theclinics.com**

It becomes more difficult to diagnosis when a patient has more than one of these conditions.[3]

The practitioner should be aware that because there are most likely different pathways to developing IC, there are probable different initial clinical characteristics and varying optimal treatment paths.

Physical Examination

Examination should target the bladder but also focus on ruling out other causes of the patient's symptoms. Minimally, providers should order urinalysis and urine culture. During pelvic examination, particular attention should be paid to whether there is any bladder tenderness. Cytology and cystoscopy should be performed if clinically indicated, such as microscopic hematuria. Clinical experience suggests a very low likelihood of missing a stone or tumor by not performing a cystoscopy in a nonsmoker under the age of 40 with a clear urinalysis.[4]

Imaging or Additional Testing

Besides history and physical examination, there are other tests that can help a provider find an accurate diagnosis. Voiding diaries of patients with IC typically show increased frequency, nocturnal frequency, and lower mean voiding volume than an average patient and may correlate with cystoscopic findings.[5] Other options to screen for IC include validated questionnaires (such as PUF [pelvic pain and urgency/frequency] or O'Leary-Sant, **Figs. 1** and **2**), a potassium sensitivity test, or an anesthetic bladder challenge, which seems useful in excluding patients with pelvic pain originating from organs other than the urinary bladder.[6] Although urodynamics are not necessarily diagnostic, they may give a provider information regarding pain with filling of the bladder, presence of detrusor overactivity, and low compliance.[7] Urinary hexosamines have been found in various studies to be significantly increased, decreased, or the same in IC/bladder pain syndrome (BPS) patients compared with controls, and, therefore, at this time cannot be relied on to be a diagnostic marker or for monitoring the condition.[4,8,9] Cystoscopy with hydrodistension (HD) can be both diagnostic and therapeutic.

A cystoscopy with HD is performed by filling the bladder with normal saline to maximal capacity at a pressure of 80 mm Hg for 1 to 2 minutes, at which point the full bladder is drained and refilled to look for glomerulations.[10] It was first reported in 1930 and at one point was considered the best option for diagnosis, but more recently it has been questioned whether it is necessary. The procedure also offers a therapeutic benefit in up to one-third of patients,[11] but this appears short-lived.[1] To prolong the therapeutic benefit, the provider needs to consider adding bladder retraining to a patient's instructions after the procedure. Cystoscopy with HD followed by bladder training (BT) produced a statistically significantly better effect than HD alone in the treatment of patients with IC. BT guidelines involved asking patient to drink water or other fluids gradually, at a speed of 150 to 20 mL/h except at mealtimes and at night. It also asked them to perform self-scheduled voids with an aim to increase the time interval and voided volume. Recommendation was given to start every 2 hours and then increase by 15-minute intervals weekly.[12] Hsieh and colleagues[1] showed that HD followed by BT, when there was good compliance, was able to produce both a good efficacy and long-term benefits. BT seems to be important for long-term remission of symptoms for patients with IC undergoing treatment (**Figs. 3** and **4**).

Summary

Cystoscopy with HD was previously considered the best option. It is currently in question as to whether this is absolutely necessary, but to date there is not a better

Patient's Name: ______________________ Today's date______________

PELVIC PAIN and URGENCY/FREQUENCY PATIENT SYMPTOM SCALE

Please circle the answer that best describes how you feel for each question.

		0	1	2	3	4	SYMPTOM SCORE	BOTHER SCORE
1	How many times do you go to the bathroom during the day?	3-6	7-10	11-14	15-19	20+		
2	a. How many times do you go to the bathroom at night?	0	1	2	3	4+		
	b. If you get up at night to go to the bathroom, does it bother you?	Never Bothers	Occasionally	Usually	Always			
3	a. Do you now or have you ever had pain or symptoms during or after sexual intercourse?	Never	Occasionally	Usually	Always			
	b. Has pain or urgency ever made you avoid sexual intercourse?	Never	Occasionally	Usually	Always			
4	Do you have pain associated with your bladder or in your pelvis (vagina, labia, lower abdomen, urethra, perineum, testes, or scrotum)?	Never	Occasionally	Usually	Always			
5	a. If you have pain, is it usually		Mild	Moderate	Severe			
	b. Does your pain bother you?	Never	Occasionally	Usually	Always			
6	Do you still have urgency after going to the bathroom?	Never	Occasionally	Usually	Always			
7	a. If you have urgency, is it usually		Mild	Moderate	Severe			
	b. Does your urgency bother you?	Never	Occasionally	Usually	Always			
8	Are you sexually active? Yes____ No____							

SYMPTOM SCORE = (1, 2a, 3a, 4, 5a, 6, 7a)	
BOTHER SCORE = (2b, 3b, 5b, 7b)	
TOTAL SCORE (Symptom Score + Bother Score) =	

Fig. 1. Pelvic pain and urgency/frequency patient symptom scale. (*Courtesy of* C. Lowell Parsons, MD; with permission. *From* Parsons CL, Dell J, Stanford EJ, et al. The prevalence of interstitial cystitis in gynecologic patients with pelvic pain, as detected by intravesical potassium sensitivity. Am J Obstet Gynecol 2002;187(5):1395–400.)

diagnostic tool. Patient history, validated questionnaires, potassium test, and ruling out other causes of pain can lead to the diagnosis, but if it is still unclear or a patient is not responding to treatment, consider performing cystoscopy with HD because this can also be therapeutic.

TREATMENT

IC is not only difficult to diagnosis but is also difficult to treat. As multiple causes or development pathways are considered for this diagnosis, it may be that eventually multiple treatment pathways will be needed. There is an argument to consider IC as a chronic pain condition rather than inflammatory bladder process.[11] As such, pain management is critical throughout diagnosis and treatment. If pain management

INTERSTITIAL CYSTITIS SYMPTOM INDEX

1.
During the past month, how often have you felt the strong need to urinate with little or no warning?

0. _______ not at all
1. _______ less than 1 time in 5
2. _______ less than half the time
3. _______ about half the time
4. _______ more than half the time
5. _______ almost always

2.
During the past month, have you had to urinate less than 2 hours after you finished urinating?

0. _______ not at all
1. _______ less than 1 time in 5
2. _______ less than half the time
3. _______ about half the time
4. _______ more than half the time
5. _______ almost always

3.
During the past month, how often did you most typically get up at night to urinate?

0. _______ never
1. _______ once
2. _______ 2 times
3. _______ 3 times
4. _______ 4 times
5. _______ 5 times
6. _______ 5 or more times

4.
During the past month, have you experienced pain or burning in your bladder?

0. _______ not at all
1. _______ once
2. _______ a few times
3. _______ fairly often
4. _______ almost always
5. _______ usually

Add the numerical values of the checked entries;
Total score _________.

INTERSTITIAL CYSTITIS PROBLEM INDEX

During the past month, how much has each of the following been a problem for you?

1. Frequent urination during the day?

0. _______ no problem
1. _______ very small problem
2. _______ small problem
3. _______ medium problem
4. _______ big problem

2. Getting up at nigth to urinate?

0. _______ no problem
1. _______ very small problem
2. _______ small problem
3. _______ medium problem
4. _______ big problem

3. Need to urinate with little warning?

0. _______ no problem
1. _______ very small problem
2. _______ small problem
3. _______ medium problem
4. _______ big problem

4. Burning, pain, discomfort, or pressure in your bladder?

0. _______ no problem
1. _______ very small problem
2. _______ small problem
3. _______ medium problem
4. _______ big problem

Add the numerical values of the check entries:
Total score _________.

Fig. 2. O'Leary/Sant voiding and pain indices. (*Adapted from* O'Leary MP, Sant GR, Fowler FJ, et al. The interstitial cystitis symptom index and problem index. Urology 1997;49(Suppl 5A): 58–63; with permission.)

offered by the primary provider is not effective, a multidisciplinary approach should be considered. The only US Food and Drug Administration (FDA) -approved treatment options for IC are pentosan polysulfate sodium (PPS) orally and intravesical dimethyl sulfoxide (DMSO), but there are many other anecdotal treatments (**Fig. 5**).

Management Goals

There is a paucity of randomized placebo-controlled trials of different therapeutic approaches, so providers are lacking an evidence-based management protocol.[13] As such, each patient's treatment should be approached uniquely with periodic re-evaluation with a standardized questionnaire to monitor objective improvement.

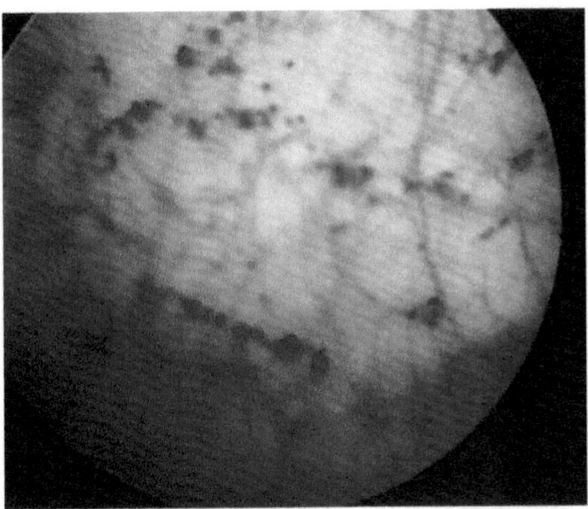

Fig. 3. Glomerulations.

Pharmacologic Strategies

Oral

The only FDA-approved oral medication to treat IC is PPS and as such this the most frequently adopted treatment.[13] It is suggested as a first-line oral medication unless there is a contraindication, such as liver disease.[4] Other alternative oral options include antihistamines (hydroxyzine, cimetidine), tricyclic antidepressants (Amitriptyline), and immune modulators.

PPS is chemically and structurally similar to glycosaminoglycans. The recommended dosage is 100 mg 3 times per day. Its therapeutic response is typically delayed however, and it can take up to 12 months before the patient responds.[14] Less than 10% of patients experience side effects, which include headache, nausea, diarrhea, dizziness, skin rash, peripheral edema, and hair loss.[15] In a systemic review of 21 randomized controlled trials, only trials for PPS had sufficient numbers to allow a pooled analysis of effect. According to a random-effects model, the pooled estimate of the effect of PPS therapy suggested benefit, with a relative risk for the patient-reported improvement in symptoms of 1.78 (95% confidence interval, 1.34–2.35).[16]

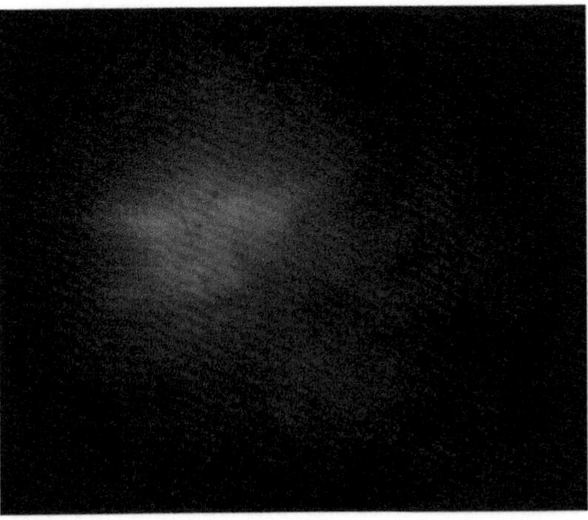

Fig. 4. Hunner ulcer.

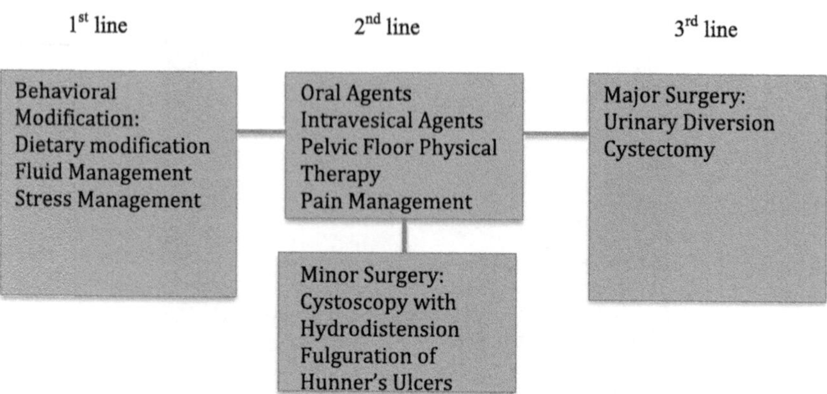

Fig. 5. Treatments of IC.

Hydroxyzine, the most commonly used antihistamine to treat IC, reduces mast cell activation and may be effective, especially in patients with allergies. In an open-label study, hydroxyzine reduced symptoms 40% overall, but it reduced them by 55% in patients who had significant allergy history.[17] Hydroxyzine also seems to work well in combination with PPS.[1] Cimetidine, a histamine H2-receptor antagonist, has been shown to be better than placebo and is inexpensive and considered relatively safe.[4]

Tricyclic antidepressants, such as amitriptyline, effectively treat neuropathic pain. Amitriptyline is typically dosed 10 to 25 mg per day, increasing dosage to increase the effect as long as side effects, including dry mouth and drowsiness, remain tolerable. Although amitriptyline is shown to be safe and effective long term, it still needs trials compared with placebo.[1,18] Amitriptyline is a good choice for a patient with unrelenting pain, due to its generalized anti-nociceptive effects.[4]

Cyclosporine A, an immune modulator, has been used for the treatment of IC off-label and has been shown to be effective. In studies, however, most patients have stopped the trial or dropped out of study because of the side effects in up to 25% of patients,[19] as the medicine may cause adverse events, such as increased creatinine or hypertension.[4]

Pain management should be considered part of treatment of this condition. Nonsteroidal anti-inflammatory drugs are thought to worsen IC/BPS symptoms in up to 10% of patients, so patients should be warned of this potential side effect before trying them; if patients are already taking these, a trial without them may be helpful to see if symptoms subside.[4]

Intravesical

Intravesical instillations for IC typically include DMSO, which is the only FDA-approved intravesical treatment, heparin, or lidocaine. Other intravesical preparations that have been tried include sodium hyaluronate, PPS, Botox, chondroitin sulfate, oxybutynin, and steroids. RTX (resiniferatoxin) and Bacillus Calmette-Guerin, which were previously used, should not be offered to patients because they do not show efficacy.[16]

DMSO is a commonly used intravesical agent for IC, and it is the only intravesical therapy since 1978 with FDA approval for the treatment of IC. DMSO works by supposed anti-inflammatory effect. It also seems to work as an analgesic and muscle relaxant and to promote collagenolysis. A typical dose of DMSO used intravesically is 50 mL of a 50% solution instilled into and retained in the bladder for 10 to 20 minutes, given 1 to 2 times a week to every few months.[1] It does, however, have many side effects including pain with the instillation, exacerbation of pain long term, and an unpleasant odor.[4]

Heparin, an anionic polyelectrolyte, is a GAG derivative. Intravesical heparin is typically dosed in 10,000 to 20,000 IU in 2 to 5 mL of solution for the duration of 1 hour, 3 times per week. Randomized control trials are needed, but Parsons and colleagues[20] showed 56% of IC patients had their symptoms relieved by heparin.

Intravesical lidocaine (1%), usually 20 to 30 mL, may be used but is typically considered short term. In a randomized trial, it was shown to have a 50% response rate when compared with placebo that had a response rate of 13%,[21] but may be typically considered short term because a long-term study only showed 8% of patients in the lidocaine group continuing to have a response at 6 months.[22] Bupivacaine should be considered because it does not require the addition of sodium bicarbonate as well as theoretically being more potent, more lipophilic, and longer lasting.[4]

Hyaluronic acid, a glycoprotein, is the traditional agent used for GAG substitution. After 6 weeks of treatment, 40 mg (50 mL) intravesical hyaluronic acid 3 times weekly produced a 52% response rate.[23] Intravesical hyaluronan has also been shown to have long-term efficacy when studied up to 5 years[24] and has also been shown to prolong the effects of HD when given intravesically weekly for 1 month after HD.[25] The challenge is to have this covered by insurance.

Intravesical oxybutynin in combination with BT has been shown to have a significant increase in bladder capacity, decrease in urinary frequency, and pain relief and did not have adverse events.[26]

Chondroitin sulfate, a glycoprotein, is a major component of the GAG layer. GAG layer replenishment is a cornerstone in the treatment of IC. A small number of randomized controlled trials confirms this treatment is favorable.[1,27]

Corticosteroids are used intravesically often in combination with other medications in a bladder cocktail for anti-inflammatory effect,[28] and therapeutic effects are particularly noticeable in patients in whom bladder biopsies show eosinophilic inflammation.[29]

PPS administrated intravesically has been shown to be effective and may produce an earlier response than the oral formulation of PPS.[29] There is a paucity of published reports using this therapy but typically 200 to 300 mg of PPS is placed in 30 to 50 mL of saline solution.[30,31]

The use of botulinum A toxin intradetrusorial injections in PBS/IC is increasing.[13] Evidence shows it may take up to 4 treatments for improvement of pain and to increase functional capacity. It does not, however, seem to benefit patients with ulcerative-type IC.[32–34] Use of intradetrusor botulinum A toxin can cause urinary retention and requires a patient to perform self-catheterization; therefore, caution should be used in any patient who has pain with catheterization.[4]

Studies on multimodal therapies and combination treatments are lacking. Those that exist are limited but size, quality, and duration of follow-up.[35]

Nonpharmacologic Strategies

Besides oral or intravesical treatments, there are other treatment approaches including physical therapy, neuromodulation, and surgery. Treatment of pelvic floor hypertonicity is an important component of treating IC. The goal of pelvic floor physical therapy in the treatment of IC/PBS, unlike that for continence, is massage of internal and external myofascial trigger points by specialized physical therapists.[36] Physical therapy techniques that involve manual or soft tissue manipulation can be used to improve symptoms in as many as 83% of patients.[37] Both global therapeutic massage and myofascial physical therapy decrease pain, urgency, and frequency ratings on the

O'Leary-Sant IC Symptom and Problem Index. When using the Global Response Assessment, which measures overall improvement with therapy, the myofascial physical therapy group was significantly more successful at 59% than the global therapeutic massage group at 26% ($P = .0012$).[38]

Sacral neuromodulation to control symptoms should be tried before surgery.[1] The IC patients would need to qualify based on frequency/urgency criteria because it is not approved by the FDA. Studies do support that it improves pain in addition to improving voiding parameters.[39] Revision rates in this patient population tend to be high and are quoted in the literature to be approximately 27% to 50%.[40–42] Posterior tibial nerve stimulation is not considered effective in the treatment of IC.[43,44] Some initial studies showed positive results in either stimulating the pudendal nerve rather than the sacral nerve or performing ultrasound-guided pudendal nerve blocks in an effort to reduce pain in these patients,[45,46] but further studies are still needed.

Minor surgery includes the previously discussed diagnostic and therapeutic cystoscopy with hydrodistention. Either fulguration and/or injection of triamcinolone into Hunner ulcers should be performed.[4,47,48] Fulguration of Hunner ulcers tend to alleviate IC symptoms and are shown to be effective when less than 25% of the bladder is involved.[49]

Major surgeries are considered a last resort for this benign condition and include bladder augmentation, urinary diversion, and cystectomy. There seems to be more complications with these procedures when performed for benign disease than for malignant disease.[50] However, major surgery is associated with good symptom relief in strictly selected patients with disabling BPS/IC, when conservative treatment has failed. Those patients with end-stage, structurally small bladders and those that lack neuropathic pain seem the best candidates.[4] Extended preoperative duration of symptoms may be a predictor for persisting pain after major surgery for BPS/IC.[51]

Self-Management Strategies

Patients can self-manage a certain amount of their symptoms by changing behaviors. They can modify their diet, alter fluid management, and work on stress management.

Nearly 90% of patients with IC can identify foods or beverages that are dietary triggers.[52] IC patients will typically find the avoidance of acidic beverages, caffeine, alcohol, chocolate, tea, soda, spicy food, citrus fruits, and artificial sweeteners helpful. Typically, if a specific food is going to worsen a patient's symptoms, it should do so within 24 hours.[4] Calcium glycerophosphate (Prelief) prevents food-related exacerbation in about 70% of patients.[53] Management of total fluid intake has also been shown to be helpful.[54]

Treating anxiety and depression as well as modifying stress is also therapeutic, because these things significantly aggravate symptoms of IC. Some patients find relief with meditation or support groups or even altering their lifestyle to make changes, including shortening work hours, choosing a less demanding workload, or exercising and practicing yoga.[1,4]

Evaluation, Adjustment, and Recurrence

One important question that remains largely unanswered is whether early detection leads to less severe disease or more easily treated disease. Warren and colleagues[55] noted when assessing prognostic factors that mild IC/PBS at baseline was the only variable that was directly associated with a mild IC/PBS endpoint.

If a patient does not respond to treatment, it is important to re-evaluate them based on objective evidence such as questionnaires as well as continuing to look for other sources of symptoms. Urinary markers may have a role in the future of monitoring this condition.

Summary/Discussion

IC is a difficult condition for both the patient and the provider. As it is a diagnosis of exclusion, it is often frustrating to find not only an accurate diagnosis but also a treatment option that is successful for the patient. It is important to target symptoms that bother the patient the most and to be flexible enough in the treatment management to move on to other options when a particular treatment is not helping. Using an objective measure of response may be helpful. There is a growing list of treatment options and, with ever-increasing research, hope for improved treatments as well as perhaps someday a cure.

REFERENCES

1. Hsieh CH, Chang WC, Huang MC, et al. Treatment of interstitial cystitis in women. Taiwan J Obstet Gynecol 2012;51(4):526–32.
2. Warren JW, Brown J, Tracy JK, et al. Evidence-based criteria for pain of interstitial cystitis/painful bladder syndrome in women. Urology 2008;71(3):444–8.
3. Bogart LM, Berry SH, Clemens JQ. Symptoms of interstitial cystitis, painful bladder syndrome and similar diseases in women: a systematic review. J Urol 2007;177(2):450–6.
4. Quillin RB, Erickson DR. Practical use of the new American Urological Association interstitial cystitis guidelines. Curr Urol Rep 2012;13(5):394–401.
5. Boudry G, Labat JJ, Riant T, et al. Validation of voiding diary for stratification of bladder pain syndrome according to the presence/absence of cystoscopic abnormalities: a two-centre prospective study. BJU Int 2013;112(2):E164–8.
6. Taneja R. Intravesical lignocaine in the diagnosis of bladder pain syndrome. Int Urogynecol J 2010;21(3):321–4.
7. Blaivas JG. Urodynamics for the evaluation of painful bladder syndrome/interstitial cystitis. J Urol 2010;184(1):16–7.
8. Buzzega D, Maccari F, Galeotti F, et al. Determination of urinary hexosamines for diagnosis of bladder pain syndrome. Int Urogynecol J 2012;23(10):1367–72.
9. Maccari F, Buzzega D, Galeotti F, et al. Fine structural characterization of chondroitin sulfate in urine of bladder pain syndrome subjects. Int Urogynecol J 2011;22(12):1581–6.
10. Hanno PM. Diagnosis of interstitial cystitis. Urol Clin North Am 1994;21:63–6.
11. Hanno P, Lin A, Nordling J, et al. Bladder Pain Syndrome Committee of the International Consultation on incontinence. Neurourol Urodyn 2010;29(1):191–8.
12. Hsieh CH, Chang WC, Huang MC, et al. Hydrodistention plus bladder training versus hydrodistention for the treatment of interstitial cystitis. Taiwan J Obstet Gynecol 2012;51(4):591–5.
13. Giannantoni A, Bini V, Dmochowski R, et al. Contemporary management of the painful bladder: a systematic review. Eur Urol 2012;61(1):29–53.
14. Hanno PM. Analysis of long-term Elmiron therapy for interstitial cystitis. Urology 1997;49(5A Suppl):93–9.
15. Jepsen JV, Sall M, Rhodes PR, et al. Long-term experience with pentosanpolysulfate in interstitial cystitis. Urology 1998;51(3):381–7.
16. Dimitrakov J, Kroenke K, Steers WD, et al. Pharmacologic management of painful bladder syndrome/interstitial cystitis: a systematic review. Arch Intern Med 2007;167(18):1922–9.
17. Theoharides TC, Sant GR. Hydroxyzine therapy for interstitial cystitis. Urology 1997;49(5A Suppl):108–10.

18. Hertle L, van Ophoven A. Long-term results of amitriptyline treatment for interstitial cystitis. Aktuelle Urol 2010;41(Suppl 1):S61–5.
19. Sairanen J, Tammela TL, Leppilahti M, et al. Cyclosporine A and pentosan polysulfate sodium for the treatment of interstitial cystitis: a randomized comparative study. J Urol 2005;174(6):2235–8.
20. Parsons C, Housley T, Schmidt JD, et al. Treatment of interstitial cystitis with intravesical heparin. Br J Urol 1994;73:504–7.
21. Parsons CL, Zupkas P, Proctor J, et al. Alkalinized lidocaine and heparin provide immediate relief of pain and urgency in patients with interstitial cystitis. J Sex Med 2012;9(1):207–12.
22. Lv YS, Zhou HL, Mao HP, et al. Intravesical hyaluronic acid and alkalinized lidocaine for the treatment of severe painful bladder syndrome/interstitial cystitis. Int Urogynecol J 2012;23(12):1715–20.
23. Van Agt S, Gobet F, Sibert L, et al. Treatment of interstitial cystitis by intravesical instillation of hyaluronic acid: a prospective study on 31 patients. Prog Urol 2011;21:218–25.
24. Engelhardt PF, Morakis N, Daha LK, et al. Long-term results of intravesical hyaluronan therapy in bladder pain syndrome/interstitial cystitis. Int Urogynecol J 2011;22(4):401–5.
25. Shao Y, Shen ZJ, Rui WB, et al. Intravesical instillation of hyaluronic acid prolonged the effect of bladder hydrodistention in patients with severe interstitial cystitis. Urology 2010;75(3):547–50.
26. Barbalias GA, Liatsikos EN, Athanasopoulos A, et al. Interstitial cystitis: bladder training with intravesical oxybutynin. J Urol 2000;163(6):1818–22.
27. Madersbacher H, van Ophoven A, van Kerrebroeck PE. GAG layer replenishment therapy for chronic forms of cystitis with intravesical glycosaminoglycans–a review. Neurourol Urodyn 2013;32(1):9–18.
28. Swift S, Chai TC, Bent AE. Painful conditions of the lower urinary tract including painful bladder syndrome. In: Bent EA, Cundiff WG, Swift ES, editors. Ostergard's urogynecology and pelvic floor dysfunction. Lippincott Williams and Wilkins; 2008. p. 106–32.
29. Sant GR, LaRock DR. Standard intravesical therapies for interstitial cystitis. Urol Clin North Am 1994;21(1):73–83.
30. Davis EL, El Khoudary SR, Talbott EO, et al. Safety and efficacy of the use of intravesical and oral pentosan polysulfate sodium for interstitial cystitis: a randomized double-blind clinical trial. J Urol 2008;179(1):177–85.
31. Bade JJ, Laseur M, Nieuwenburg A, et al. A placebo-controlled study of intravesical pentosanpolysulphate for the treatment of interstitial cystitis. Br J Urol 1997;79(2):168–71.
32. Kuo HC. Repeated intravesical onabotulinumtoxinA injections are effective in treatment of refractory interstitial cystitis/bladder pain syndrome. Int J Clin Pract 2013;67(5):427–34.
33. Lee CL, Kuo HC. Intravesical botulinum toxin a injections do not benefit patients with ulcer type interstitial cystitis. Pain Physician 2013;16(2):109–16.
34. Kuo HC. Repeated onabotulinumtoxin-a injections provide better results than single injection in treatment of painful bladder syndrome. Pain Physician 2013;16(1):E15–23.
35. French LM, Bhambore N. Interstitial cystitis/painful bladder syndrome. Am Fam Physician 2011;83(10):1175–81.
36. Elliott CS, Payne CK. Interstitial cystitis and the overlap with overactive bladder. Curr Urol Rep 2012;13(5):319–26.

37. Weiss JM. Pelvic floor myofascial trigger points: manual therapy for interstitial cystitis and the urgency-frequency syndrome. J Urol 2001;166(6):2226–31.
38. FitzGerald MP, Payne CK, Lukacz ES, et al. Randomized multicenter clinical trial of myofascial physical therapy in women with interstitial cystitis/painful bladder syndrome and pelvic floor tenderness. J Urol 2012;187(6):2113–8.
39. Ghazwani YQ, Elkelini MS, Hassouna MM. Efficacy of sacral neuromodulation in treatment of bladder pain syndrome: long-term follow-up. Neurourol Urodyn 2011;30(7):1271–5.
40. Gajewski JB, Al-Zahrani AA. The long-term efficacy of sacral neuromodulation in the management of intractable cases of bladder pain syndrome: 14 years of experience in one centre. BJU Int 2011;107(8):1258–64.
41. Marinkovic SP, Gillen LM, Marinkovic CM. Minimum 6-year outcomes for interstitial cystitis treated with sacral neuromodulation. Int Urogynecol J 2011;22(4):407–12.
42. Powell CR, Kreder KJ. Long-term outcomes of urgency-frequency syndrome due to painful bladder syndrome treated with sacral neuromodulation and analysis of failures. J Urol 2010;183(1):173–6.
43. Zhao J, Nordling J. Posterior tibial nerve stimulation in patients with intractable interstitial cystitis. BJU Int 2004;94(1):101–4.
44. Zhao J, Bai J, Zhou Y, et al. Posterior tibial nerve stimulation twice a week in patients with interstitial cystitis. Urology 2008;71(6):1080–4.
45. Lean LL, Hegarty D, Harmon D. Analgesic effect of bilateral ultrasound-guided pudendal nerve blocks in management of interstitial cystitis. J Anesth 2012; 26(1):128–9.
46. Peters KM, Feber KM, Bennett RC. A prospective, single-blind, randomized crossover trial of sacral vs pudendal nerve stimulation for interstitial cystitis. BJU Int 2007;100(4):835–9.
47. Cox M, Klutke JJ, Klutke CG. Assessment of patient outcomes following submucosal injection of triamcinolone for treatment of Hunner's ulcer subtype interstitial cystitis. Can J Urol 2009;16(2):4536–40.
48. Hanno PM, Burks DA, Clemens JQ, et al. AUA guideline for the diagnosis and treatment of interstitial cystitis/bladder pain syndrome. J Urol 2011;185(6):2162–70.
49. Hillelsohn JH, Rais-Bahrami S, Friedlander JI, et al. Fulguration for Hunner ulcers: long-term clinical outcomes. J Urol 2012;188(6):2238–41.
50. Nickel JC. Editorial comment. Urology 2013;82(4):833 [discussion: 833].
51. Andersen AV, Granlund P, Schultz A, et al. Long-term experience with surgical treatment of selected patients with bladder pain syndrome/interstitial cystitis. Scand J Urol Nephrol 2012;46(4):284–9.
52. Friedlander JI, Shorter B, Moldwin RM. Diet and its role in interstitial cystitis/bladder pain syndrome (IC/BPS) and comorbid conditions. BJU Int 2012; 109(11):1584–91.
53. Howard F. When treating interstitial cystitis, treat all sources of pain. OBG Management 2010;22(7):33–49.
54. Foster HE Jr, Hanno PM, Nickel JC, et al. Effect of amitriptyline on symptoms in treatment naive patients with interstitial cystitis/painful bladder syndrome. J Urol 2010;183(5):1853–8.
55. Warren JW, Clauw DJ, Langenberg P. Prognostic factors for recent-onset interstitial cystitis/painful bladder syndrome. BJU Int 2013;111(3 Pt B):E92–7.

Myofascial Pelvic Pain

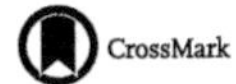

Theresa Monaco Spitznagle, PT, DPT, MHS, WCS[a,*],
Caitlin McCurdy Robinson, PT, DPT[b]

KEYWORDS

• Pelvic pain • Myofascial pain syndrome • Somatovisceral convergence

KEY POINTS

- Myofascial pelvic pain should be considered in women seeking medical care for pain in the pelvic region.
- Although the cause is unknown, consideration of the neural input, regional pelvic structures, and specific muscular demands may explain causes of myofascial pain.
- Myofascial pain is diagnosed by the presence of pain with palpation of muscle and connective tissue in the region of pain.
- Conservative interventions to consider for myofascial pelvic pain include soft-tissue mobilization, biofeedback, electrical stimulation, correction of movement impairments with therapeutic exercise and activities, and dry needling.

INTRODUCTION

Individuals with pelvic pain commonly present with complaints of pain located anywhere below the umbilicus radiating to the top of their thighs or genital region.[1] Because of the location of pelvic pain, women seek care with their gynecologist believing that their ovaries or uterus to be the source of their discomfort.[2–5] Pelvic pain, however, is multifactorial, encompassing multiple systems, including gastroenterologic, urologic, gynecologic, oncologic, musculoskeletal, and psychological.[6,7] The association of organ disease with pelvic region pain is high.[3,6,8] It is estimated that between 25% and 40% of women receiving laparoscopic surgery for pelvic pain do not have an obvious structural diagnosis.[9,10]

Myofascial pain is a common condition found in individuals seeking medical care.[11] Myofascial pelvic pain, thus, is part of the algorithm for determining the source of pelvic pain. The somatovisceral convergence[12] that occurs within the pelvic region exemplifies why examination of not only the organs but also the muscles, connective tissue (fascia), and neurologic input to the region should be performed for women with pelvic pain (**Table 1**). Although the mechanism for development of myofascial pelvic pain is

---

The authors have nothing to disclose.
[a] Program in Physical Therapy, Washington University School of Medicine, 4444 Forest Park, Box 8502, St Louis, MO 63108-2212, USA; [b] Sullivan Physical Therapy, Austin, TX 78750, USA
* Corresponding author.
E-mail address: spitznaglet@wustl.edu

Obstet Gynecol Clin N Am 41 (2014) 409–432
http://dx.doi.org/10.1016/j.ogc.2014.04.003 obgyn.theclinics.com
0889-8545/14/$ – see front matter

Table 1
Somatovisceral conditions

Viscera Condition	Somatic Condition	Reference
Bone tuberculosis	Pain to touch in soft tissues surrounding the coccyx and L gluteal region	70
Capsaicin-stimulated gut pain	Skin temperature increase and increased blood flow in abdominal wall	71
Cardiac ischemia	Chest wall tenderness to touch	72
Endometriosis	Myofascial trigger point pain, including the abdomen, perineum, levator ani and obturator internus muscles	73
Gall bladder disease	Shoulder pain Trigger points in the right upper quadrant of the abdomen, tropic changes of the skin	74–76
Migraine	Cervical muscle trigger points, cutaneous allodynia	77,78
Pneumothoracic	Limited range of motion in neck	79
Pustulotic arthro-osteitis	Pain to touch in gluteal region	80
Splenic rupture	Pain to touch along subcostal margin	81
Ureterolithiasis	Flank pain, trigger points in dermatome pattern	82

not clearly understood, consideration of this condition early in the management of pelvic pain may be paramount to avoidance of unnecessary procedures.[13]

Definitions

Myofascial pain syndrome is classically described as a myalgia condition with local and referred pain patterns.[14,15] The perception of pain is regulated by both the central and peripheral nervous systems.[16] Thus, the term myofascial pain is inherently confusing. The simple definition, pain that arises from muscle and fascia, ignores the contribution of the nervous system to muscle function. Another point of confusion in the definition of myofascial pain is that muscles have a functional role related to movement. The functional state of a muscle depends on moderators of the movement system. Movement system is defined as a physiologic system that functions to produce motion of the body as a whole or of its component parts.[17,18] Thus, consideration of the component parts of muscle performance including architecture and muscle performance (length, strength, motor control) should be included in defining the impairments associate with myofascial pain. Trigger points, palpable nodules that are tender to touch that refer pain beyond the local tissue and are commonly found in taut bands of muscle fibers, are consistently associated with myofascial pain.[14] However, latent trigger points do exist that are not painful to touch.[19] Some investigators believe that pain to touch of the connective and muscle in a region regardless of the presence of a trigger point to be myofascial pain.[15] Muscle does not function in isolation; thus, a more detailed definition of myofascial pain has been proposed, which includes pain to touch of a muscle, local and referred; presence of an active trigger point; loss of range of motion of a specific muscle or fascia associated with the muscle; and autonomic dysfunction including cellular and physiologic changes.[20] For the purposes of this article, the following definition is used for myofascial pain: a complex form of neuromuscular dysfunction consisting of motor and sensory abnormalities involving both the peripheral and central nervous systems.[21]

ETIOLOGY

The cause of pelvic floor muscle pain is not fully understood. There are several theories that are being proposed and have been investigated in other regions of the body. These theories include a metabolic imbalance at the peripheral tissue,[20,21] centralized pain phenomenon,[15,16] and neuromuscular microtrauma that is the result of sustained positions and movement impairments of the lumbopelvic region.[7,22,23] Each theory is briefly reviewed to illustrate the issues associated with myofascial pain.

METABOLIC IMBALANCE

Gerwin and colleagues[20] propose that the altered activity of the motor end plate is part of the mechanism that underlies myofascial pain. The theory suggests that an increase in acetylcholine at the receptor site changes the biochemical response to muscle activity associated with spasm of a muscle, causing an increase in muscle fiber activity at the site of a trigger point.[20] This theory is an expansion of the original ideas of Janet Travel and David Simons, which postulated that trigger points are a key source of myofascial pain.[24] Nociceptive pain is proposed to be present because of microscopic muscle damage from muscle-contraction-induced hypoxia, alternation in pH, and a release of muscle metabolites, including adenosine triphosphate, bradykinin, 5-hydrozytryptamine, prostaglandins, cytokines, calcitonin gene-related peptide, and potassium.[20] The muscle soreness common in eccentric muscle exercise exemplifies this type of pain.[25] There still remains limited evidence to support this theory. However, Shah and Gilliams,[21] using microdialysis to sample the local substances surrounding active trigger point found differences in active painful regions of a muscle compared with nonpainful regions. Although this theory provides a possible explanation for the peripheral tissue changes that are thought to occur in myofascial pain, Gerwin and colleagues[20] recognize that with peripheral changes that are sustained over time, there most likely is centralized change in the neural control of the peripheral tissues.

CENTRALIZED PAIN

Recognition that a muscle is painful to touch provides only the starting point for understanding why myofascial pain is present. Pain research indicates the need to consider not only the peripheral but also centralized changes of the entire nervous system.[16] Kuner[16] proposes that there is a central mechanism of pathologic pain and that disease-induced (neural) plasticity can occur at both structural and functional levels (of the nervous system) manifesting in changes in individual molecules, synapses, cellular function, and network activity. This theory suggests that there is a perpetuation of pain to touch, which occurs after trauma to the muscle by means of a neural adaptive response. The sensation of pain is perceived centrally after a network of neural fibers transmits a signal through the spinal canal to the brain. It is thought that there are changes in glial cell proliferation and neuronal loss at the spinal level, as well as a central sensitization, which can explain the awareness of nociceptive triggers distal to the original region of injury or in adjacent tissues. Thus, because of this neural adaptation, the longer an individual has pain the more likely it will persist.[16]

MOVEMENT

Myofascial pain in other regions has been attributed to overuse injuries and subsequent muscle length changes.[26,27] That the pelvic floor musculature is susceptible to the development of myofascial pain has been attributed to unique functional demands of this muscle.[28] Consideration of the movement demands of the region is paramount to understanding the underlying mechanism for the development of pain.[17] Correction of alignment and movement impairments has been found to reduce or abolish musculoskeletal pain in the abdomen,[29] back,[30–32] knee,[33] neck,[34,35] and shoulder.[36] Thus, it is logical to consider correction of movement impairments of the lumbopelvic region in women with myofascial pelvic pain.

The first step in understanding the function of a muscle is to consider its architecture.[37] The architecture of pelvic floor muscle has only been investigated in a limited fashion. Tuttle and colleagues,[38] performed a series of fresh dissections to describe the architecture of the pelvic floor muscles. Key findings included (1) significant differences in fiber length across each region of the pelvic floor musculature (coccygeus = 5.29 ± 0.32 cm, iliococcygeus = 7.55 ± 0.46 cm, pubovisceral = 10.45 ± 0.67 cm), (2) predominantly connective tissue in the region of the iliococcygeus muscle, and (3) sarcomere lengths shorter than other skeletal muscles (ie, transverse abdominis = 2.7 μm compared with coccygeus = 2.05 ± 0.02 μm, iliococcygeus = 2.02 ± 0.02 μm, pubovisceral = 2.07 ± 0.01 μm). These findings support the concept that the pelvic floor muscle has regional functional demands. The pubovisceral muscle with the longer muscle fibers is more likely to lengthen in response to internal loads (parturition, defecation, and gait). The iliococcygeus muscle has a supportive function and thus an increase in connective tissue. Lastly, all regions of the pelvic floor muscle can produce more force when stretched because of their shortened sarcomere lengths.[38] Tuttle goes on to suggest that "It is possible that pelvic floor muscle contraction could allow some of the load to be borne by the bony pelvic ring or through compensatory muscle actions of the obturator internus muscle."[38] Thus, it is logical to consider that if there is an impairment in any one of the contributing components of the levator ani muscle function (muscle, nerve, connective tissue) and/or the functional demand increases (run a half marathon, bronchitis, prolonged birth of child, or constipation), the pelvic floor muscle may develop a myofascial pain syndrome. Tuttle also noted that typical pressure demands on the pelvic floor muscles for functional activities like coughing and jumping far exceeds the architectural function of the pelvic floor musculature.[38] This provides one possible explanation for the development of intra-abdominal pressure-related muscle pain.

CLINICAL FINDINGS

Physical Examination

To determine the presence of myofascial pain in the pelvic floor muscles, it has been suggested to perform a physical examination of the local tissues.[7,28] Recognition of a palpable nodule or tight band of tissue that reproduces a twitch response, as well as local and/or referred pain to the pelvic organs or surrounding tissues, has been the standard for identification of myofascial pain.[24] There have been several attempts to establish reliability of the physical examination with mixed results.[39–43] Unfortunately, palpation techniques are varied and succinct descriptions lacking. It has been suggested that tester training with a pressure algometer, which provides feedback to the examiners on the amount of pressure during palpation, could make the examination more reliable.[44–46]

The stability of myofascial pelvic pain has not been established. Simply examining the patient in one instance may effectively be providing feedback to the nervous system and subsequently change the sensation of pain. Thus, if the patient's position changed or there was a variation in the patient's emotional state, there could be more or less pain noted on examination. In addition, it is unclear how much myofascial pain varies in relationship to other organ disease. For example, it is currently unknown if individuals with interstitial cystitis having a flare of bladder pain also get a flare of myofascial pelvic pain. More research in this area is needed.

Lastly, the pelvic floor musculature does not function in isolation but is a component of the movement associated with the lumbopelvic region. Extrapelvic structures are consistently included in the physical examination process for pelvic region pain.[22,23] Inclusion of palpation and movement testing of the spine, pelvis, and hip aides in providing insight into contributing factors and specific functional activities that may be causing a myofascial pelvic syndrome.

Diagnostic Tests

At present, there are some emerging diagnostic tests available to determine the presence of a trigger point in a muscle. First, as previously mentioned, Shah and colleagues[21,47] were able to use microdialysis to assess microscopic substances associated with muscle metabolism. Imaging of the muscle via magnetic resonance elastography has been executed.[48] Chen and colleagues[48] demonstrated differences in muscle across 2 subjects undergoing magnetic resonance elastography. Ultrasound imaging has been used to objectively demonstrate the presence of a trigger point and describe the vascular changes in the region of the tissues.[49–53] Finally, Maher and colleagues[54] measured the shear modulus of a palpable trigger point using ultrasound shear wave elastography and demonstrated tissue changes after dry needling. The use of new technology for imaging and microdialysis may in the future provide more objective measures of trigger points associated with myofascial pain. However, at this time, palpation remains the best method for diagnosis.

TREATMENT

Interventions most commonly prescribed for myofascial pelvic pain are designed to address pain and range of motion loss of the local and regional tissues (muscle/fascia, nerve, and joints). There is moderate evidence to support the use of manual techniques, when combined with other physical therapy techniques such as exercise, biofeedback, and electrical stimulation to improve pain severity, bowel, bladder, and sexual function in both adult men and women with myofascial pelvic pain.[55–67] Although myofascial pelvic pain has been more commonly associated with women, at present more men than women have been studied who have this condition (see **Table 2** for details on articles). Manual manipulations of the tissues include trigger point release,[55–58,60,62,64–66,68] massage,[57,60,64–66] and stretching[63,67] and are applied directly to the pelvic floor musculature. A trigger point release is an internal or external digital pressure applied to trigger points in the pelvic floor/levator ani muscles. Manual interventions are commonly combined, including elements of trigger point release, massage, and stretching.[60,64–67,69] Common interventions that are used in addition to the manual techniques include biofeedback,[63–67] electrical stimulation,[63,64,66] dilator usage,[63–65] exercise/stretching,[58–60,62–67] and dry needling.[54] Corrective exercises aid in retraining movement and reduce mechanical stress on the tissues potentially affecting both the peripheral and central adaptations that perpetuate chronic pain. Inclusion of psychological services for cognitive behavioral interventions including instruction on relaxation techniques are also warranted in this population.[57–60,68]

Table 2
What are the effects of manual physical therapy techniques on function and pain severity in patients with myofascial pelvic pain?

		Subject Characteristics				Intervention Details			Results				
									Function				
Author and Year	LOER, Study Type, PEDro Rating	N, Sex	Age (y)	Medical Dx	Duration of Sx	Frequency and Duration	Manual PT Techniques	Additional or Comparative Techniques	Bowel	Bladder	Sexual	Pain	Reviewers' Conclusions
Fitzgerald et al,[56] 2012	1b:RCT, single blind RCT, 7/10	81, ♂: 0, ♀: 81	43 med (18–77)	• IC	>3 mo, ≤3 y	• 10 visits • 1 h • 1x/wk	MPT group: • Tissue manipulation: ab wall, back, buttocks, thighs • CTM: (B) from T10-popliteal crease, (B) thighs from knee up; ab wall from suprapubic rim to anterior costal cartilages • TPR: internal and external Performed until texture change was noted	Additive techniques: • PFM drops to length the PF • HEP: individualized (no Kegels) Comparison group: 1. GTM: 1 h traditional full-body Western massage (effleurage, petrissage, friction, tapotement, vibration, and kneading) to UE, LE, trunk, gluteals, abdomen, head, and neck	N/A	Urgency Likert: MPT: • Baseline: 6.1 • 12 wk: 3.9 GTM: • Baseline: 6.0 • 12 wk: 4.7 Freq Likert: MPT: • Baseline: 6.5 • 12 wk: 4.3 GTM: • Baseline: 6.2 • 12 wk: 4.9 24-h Freq: MPT: • Baseline: 13.6 • 12 wk: 11.6 GTM: • Baseline: 12.4 • 12 wk: 11.1	FSFI 2000: MPT: • Baseline: 18.7 • 12 wk: 20.5 GTM: • Baseline: 20.7 • 12 wk: 22.2	NPRS: MPT: • Baseline: 6.5 • 12 wk: 3.8 GTM: • Baseline: 5.8 • 12 wk: 4.3	Strong Evidence to suggest that: • Manual PT techniques may produce improvements in pain, sexual function, or urinary function (urge/freq), but are not more effective than GTM • Statistically significant improvement in pts' perception of their overall symptoms (GRA score) compared with GTM Other: • Over 50% of pts receiving manual techniques may report an adverse event, primarily pain (64%), but was

										ICSI: MPT: • Baseline: 11.9 • 12 wk: 8.6 GTM: • Baseline: 11.4 • 12 wk: 9.3 ICPI: MPT: • Baseline: 10.5 • 12 wk: 6.9 GTM: • Baseline: 10.7 • 12 wk: 8.3			not statistically significant compared with the GTM group
Olszewski,[65] 2012	4: Case study, pretest/posttest, 2/10	1, ♂: 0, ♀: 1	39	• Vestibulodynia • SUI	≥8 y	• 9 visits • 45 min • 3 mo	• TPR (1–2 min) to discomfort, but not pain • Thiele massage: 10 reps (3- to 6- and 9- to 6-o'clock positions) • Dilator: 5 s around the introitus at each segment	Additive techniques: • BF (including dilator for relaxation) • Lower ab/TA exercises • Nutrition Comparison groups: N/A	Pt report of bearing down: • Baseline: bearing down during 2/3 bowel movement, would bear down >25% of the time during bowel movement • 5th visit: no straining Pt report of stool quality:	Pt report of episodes of incontinence: • Baseline: 1 episode per 3 d • 4th visit: 0 episodes Pt report of hesitancy • Baseline: NA • 5 sessions: no longer having hesitancy	N/A	NPRS: External TPs: • Baseline: 4–6/10 • 9th visit: 0/10 Internal TPs: • Baseline: 8/10 • 9th visit: 2/10 Tampon insertion: • Baseline: NA • 5th visit: 0/10 Pt report of pain c/intercourse: • Baseline: 7/10 pain c/initial penetration	Weak Evidence that: • Individualized PT tx including manual techniques may improve: urinary continence, pain c/intercourse/tampon insertion, tenderness to palpation • PT including nutrition education may help with stool quality • Individualized PT treatment

(*continued on next page*)

Table 2
(*continued*)

Author and Year	LOER, Study Type, PEDro Rating	Subject Characteristics: N, Sex	Subject Characteristics: Age (y)	Subject Characteristics: Medical Dx	Subject Characteristics: Duration of Sx	Intervention Details: Frequency and Duration	Intervention Details: Manual PT Techniques	Intervention Details: Additional or Comparative Techniques	Results: Function: Bowel	Results: Function: Bladder	Results: Function: Sexual	Results: Pain	Reviewers' Conclusions
									• Baseline: hard stool • 5th visit: softer stool			and 5/10 during intercourse • 7th visit: 50% less pain with intercourse • 8th visit: 0/10	may improve movement pattern during defecation, but because the manual techniques were not applied intrarectally cannot associate the improvement c/manual techniques
Anderson et al,[62] 2011	2b: Individual cohort study, pretest/ posttest, 2/10	116, ♂: 116, ♀: 0	48 med (19–80)	• Prostatitis • Isolated orchialgia • Pudendal neuralgia	4.8 y	PT (TPR): • 5 d, consecutively • 30–60 min	• TPR: 4 kg/cm^2 and instruction on self-performance	Additive techniques: • Psych: PRT training • HEP: instructed how to stretch Comparison group: N/A	N/A	NIH-CPSI urinary: • Baseline: 4 • Post-tx: 2 PPSS Urinary: • Baseline: 10.5 • Post-tx: 6	PPSS sexual: • Baseline: 5 • Post-tx: 3	NIH-CPSI pain: • Baseline: 12 • Post-tx: 9 PPSS VAS (1-10 scale): • Baseline: 4 • Post-tx: 3	Moderate Evidence for: • Significant improvement in bladder/sexual fxn outcome measure scores, pain, and pt's perception of sx (GRA) when combined c/PRT • Possible maintenance of gains at 6-mo f/u; hard to determine b/c only reassessed total NIH-CPSI score Other:

													• Not feasible for clinical application • Good pt compliance c/relaxation tapes (78%) and relaxation exercises (62%) following tx
Figures et al,[66] 2010	4: Case series, retrospective chart review, 2/10	5, ♂:0, ♀: 5	52 ($\bar{x}$) (20–80)	• IC • Urinary retention • UUI • Levator spasm	13 y	• 7 visits ($\bar{x}$) • 10–16 wk	• Internal/ external manual therapy (NOS) • Myofascial release (TPR) • Dilator: internal massage and desensitization	Additive techniques: • Bladder training (positioning) • PFM: contract/relax • BF • Stretching: ab and hip flexors • Nutrition • HEP: NOS Comparison groups: N/A	N/A	Self-catheterization: • Baseline: 3 required self-catheterization • Post-tx: 2 no longer needed to perform and 1 DEC frequency to 3x/d (baseline: 12x/d)	N/A	NPRS: • Baseline: 5.3 • Post-tx: 1.3	Weak Evidence that: • Individualized PT tx including manual PT techniques may DEC need for self-catheterization and DEC pain Other: • No definition of techniques • No definitive freq/duration
Gentilcore-Saulnier,[63] 2010	2b: Individual cohort study, prospective cohort, pretest/ posttest for treatment group only, 3/10	22 (11 ctrls), ♂: 0, ♀: 22	22 ($\bar{x}$)	• PVD	4 y ($\bar{x}$)	• 8 visits • 60–75 min/visit • 12 wk ($\bar{x}$) • 15–20 min of manual • 30 s/ technique	• Stretching: at 5-, 6-, and 7-o'clock positions progressing from fingers extended to PIPs flexed to 90° and increasing from 1 to 2 fingers width	Additive techniques: • Dilator insertion • BF • E-stim: using Femiscan probe (Biomation, Almonte, ON, Canada) and Danmeter Elpha II 3000 electric stimulator (Biomation, Almonte, ON, Canada)	N/A	N/A	N/A	NPRS: Intravaginal palpation: • Baseline: 2.3 • Post-tx: 0.36 Tolerance to dilator: • Baseline: N/A • Post-tx: 91% were able to insert ½ the length of D3 dilator c/pain of ≤4/10 Pressure pain sensitivity:	Moderate Evidence for: • Statistically significant DEC in pain c/intravaginal palpation • Improved tolerance to dilator insertion, responsiveness to pain, and pressure pain sensitivity

(continued on next page)

Table 2
(continued)

Author and Year	LOER, Study Type, PEDro Rating	Subject Characteristics: N, Sex	Subject Characteristics: Age (y)	Subject Characteristics: Medical Dx	Subject Characteristics: Duration of Sx	Intervention Details: Frequency and Duration	Intervention Details: Manual PT Techniques	Intervention Details: Additional or Comparative Techniques	Results: Function: Bowel	Results: Function: Bladder	Results: Function: Sexual	Results: Pain	Reviewers' Conclusions
							• Soft-tissue mobilization	• HEP: PFM contractions and dilator insertion Comparison groups: N/A; control group only used at baseline to evaluate differences in baseline characteristics				• Baseline: N/A • Post-tx: 37% INC in amount of pressure required to elicit pain	
Chiarioni et al,[59] 2010	1b:RCT, Stratified randomization, single blind RCT, 7/10	157, ♂:81,[a] ♀:76[a]	42[a] (18–70)	• Chronic or recurrent rectal pain	1.33 y[a] (16.6 mo[a])	• 9 visits • 30–45 min • 3x/wk	• Intrarectal massage: pressure to tolerance rotating from side to side 4–6x → 20x. • Taught to perform 2x/d	Additive techniques: • Counseling performed during sessions • Warm sitz bath before home performance of massage Comparison groups: 1. BF: 5, 30 min visits, 1x/wk	Balloon expulsion (% success): BF: • Baseline: 39[a] • 1-mo f/u: 91.5[a] • 3-mo f/u: 90[a] EGS: • Baseline: 34[a] • 1-mo f/u: 58[a] • 3-mo f/u: 59.5[a]	N/A	N/A	VAS: • Authors reported significant changes in average VAS rating of pain in the BF group > ECS > massage in those with highly likely LAS # Days/mo c/pain: • DEC significantly in BF group > massage or EGS	Strong Evidence that: • BF can produce statistically significant improvements in ave weekly rectal pain intensity for up to 6 mo, but only in those c/highly likely dx of LAS, but massage does not • Massage can produce

								2. EGS: 9, 30- to 45-min visits, 3x/wk	Massage: • Baseline: 52.5[a] • 1-mo f/u: 62.5[a] • 3-mo f/u: 65.5[a]				statistically significant improvements in defecation but only in those c/highly likely dx of LAS • The effects of BF on defeca-tion are > massage c/statistically significant amounts and were found effective in those c/highly likely and possible dx of LAS Other: • Specific data tables for many of the outcome measures were not provided • DEC adherence to self-performance of intrarectal massage as time lapsed
Van Alstyne et al,[58] 2010	4: Case series, pretest/ posttest, 2/10	2, ♂: 2, ♀: 0	49 ($\bar{x}$) (45–53)	• CP • IBS	>1.25 y, >3 y (respec-tively)	• 2x/wk • 30–60 s of TPR	• TPR: ab and transrectal regions, pressure to pt's tolerance level	Additive techniques: • Ther ex: hip ROM, postural training • PRT	N/A	NIH-CPSI urinary: • Baseline: 2.5 • Post-tx: 2	Modified PPSS: • Baseline: 3 • Post-tx: 1.5 (pt 1: 0; pt 2: 3—no change)	NPRS: • Baseline: 8.5 • Post-tx: (pt 1: 0/10-9 point DEC; pt 2: 4/10-4 point DEC) • 1-y f/u: 0 NIH-CPSI pain:	Weak Evidence for: • Clinically significant (6 point) change in pain on NIH-CPSI

(*continued on next page*)

Table 2
(*continued*)

Author and Year	LOER, Study Type, PEDro Rating	Subject Characteristics: N, Sex	Age (y)	Medical Dx	Duration of Sx	Intervention Details: Frequency and Duration	Manual PT Techniques	Additional or Comparative Techniques	Results: Function: Bowel	Bladder	Sexual	Pain	Reviewers' Conclusions
								• MHP to lower ab, (15 min) • HEP: aerobic exercise, lower ab strengthening, hip stretching, and lumbar extension exercise Comparison groups: N/A			• 1-y f/u: pts denied pain c/ intercourse	• Baseline: 15 • Post-tx: 6	Other: • Long-term improvements > short term in pain and fxn. Therefore, may have been outside factors not tx • Long-term effects were the same regardless of whether performed by PT or by pt's spouse
Fitzgerald et al,[57] 2009	1b:RCT, single-blind RCT, 7/10	47, ♂: 23, ♀: 24	43[b] ($\bar{x}$) (22–76)	• CP • IC	>3 mo, ≤3 y	• 10 visits • 1 h/visit • 1x/wk Initially: ½ time spent on external tissues, progressed to more time spent on internal	• Tissue manipulation: ab wall, back, buttocks, thighs • CTM: (B) from T10-popliteal crease, (B) thighs from knee up; ab wall from suprapubic rim to anterior costal cartilages • TPR: internal	Additive techniques: • PFM drops to length the PF • HEP: individualized (No Kegels) Comparison group: 1. GTM	N/A	IC Urgency severity Score: MPT: • Baseline: 6.8 • Post-tx: 4.0 GTM: • Baseline: 6.7 • Post-tx: 6.3 Frequency severity score: MPT: • Baseline: 7.2 • Post-tx: 3.5 GTM:	IC FSFI-2000: MPT: • Baseline: 21.3 • Post-tx: 25.3 GTM: • Baseline: 18.4 • Post-tx: 21.7 CP SHIM: MPT: • Baseline: 18.8 • Post-tx: 16.4 GTM: • Baseline: 17.1	IC NPRS: MPT: • Baseline: 6.8 • Post-tx: 4.2 GTM: • Baseline: 6.7 • Post-tx: 5.9 CP NIH-CPSI pain (0–21): MPT: • Baseline: 14.2 • Post-tx: 8.0 GTM: • Baseline: 12.7	Strong Evidence that: • MPT produces statistically significant improvements in pts perception of sx (GRA), NPRS score, and urinary fxn (urge/freq) in those c/IC or CP, but only better than GTM in ICPI and ICSI scores; MPT only better than GTM at improving outcome measure scores but not specific

		and external Performed until texture change was noted	• Baseline: 7.6 • Post-tx: 6.8 ICSI: MPT: • Baseline: 13.0 • Post-tx: 8.1 GTM: • Baseline: 12.8 • Post-tx: 12.9 ICPI: MPT: • Baseline: 12.1 • Post-tx: 7.3 GTM: • Baseline: 11.5 • Post-tx: 10.8 CP NIH-CPSI urinary MPT: • Baseline: 8.9 • Post-tx: 5.0 GTM: • Baseline: 4.6 • Post-tx: 3.9 ICSI: MPT:	• Post-tx: 18.6	• Post-tx: 8.2	symptom severity • MPT may improve sexual fxn, per outcome measure scores, in those with IC, but not those with CP Other: • Men c/CP were different at baseline in regards to the ICPI and ICSI scores than those with IC →could be that those with higher scores have more tx effect than those with lower starting scores or may be effect on men vs women • High % of adverse events in those receiving MPT (52%) v GTM (21%)

(continued on next page)

Table 2
(*continued*)

Author and Year	LOER, Study Type, PEDro Rating	Subject Characteristics: N, Sex	Subject Characteristics: Age (y)	Subject Characteristics: Medical Dx	Subject Characteristics: Duration of Sx	Intervention Details: Frequency and Duration	Intervention Details: Manual PT Techniques	Intervention Details: Additional or Comparative Techniques	Results: Function: Bowel	Results: Function: Bladder	Results: Function: Sexual	Results: Pain	Reviewers' Conclusions
										• Baseline: 11.3 • Post-tx: 6.7 GTM: • Baseline: 5.6 • Post-tx: 4.3 ICPI: MPT: • Baseline: 10.4 • Post-tx: 5.4 GTM: • Baseline: 3.8 • Post-tx: 3.5			
Goldfinger et al,[64] 2009	2b: Individual cohort study, pretest/posttest, 2/10	13, ♂: 0, ♀: 13	23 ($\bar{x}$) (19–31)	• PVD	3.7 y ($\bar{x}$)	• 8 visits • 60–75 min/visit • Over 10–19 wk	• TPR • Massage (progression of techniques included increased number of fingers 1→2 and increasing pressure)	Additive techniques: • BF: Femiscan probe • E-stim: 5–12 min c/Femiscan probe and Danmeter Elpha II 3000 • Dilator: INC diameter from 3.3 to 4.0 cm	N/A	N/A	FSFI: • Baseline: 20.15 • Post-tx: 24.60 • 3-mo f/u: 25.81 SS-SE: • Baseline: 17.54 • Post-tx: 14.31 # Monthly intercourse attempts: • Baseline: 4.46	Vestibular pain index: • Baseline: 5.23 • Post-tx: 2.06 Pain threshold: • Baseline: 49.46 • Post-tx: 134.61 Intercourse pain intensity: • Baseline: 6.73 • Post-tx: 2.23 • 3-mo f/u: 2.27 Intercourse pain/unpleasantness: • Baseline: 6.77 • Post-tx: 2.14 • 3-mo f/u: 2.50	Moderate Evidence supporting: • Manual techniques when added to BF, e-stim, dilator, and HEP can produce significant improvements in pain thresholds, vestibular pain index, intercourse unpleasantness, intercourse pain intensity,

								• HEP: NOS Comparison groups: N/A			• Post-tx: 3.23 • 3-mo f/u: 5.0	% Painful intercourse attempts: • Baseline: 97.27 • Post-tx: 54.09 • 3-mo f/u: 39.91	and % painful intercourse attempts • Limited long-term effects, as changes in intercourse pain and unpleasantness declined from post-tx to 3-mo f/u • Overall, significant improvement in FSFI score, specifically in satisfaction and pain • No significant effect in SS-SE scores Other: • Pain threshold improvement may be secondary to desensitization techniques
Anderson et al,[68] 2006	4: Case series, pretest/posttest, 2/10	146, ♂: 146, ♀: 0	42 ($\bar{x}$) (18–77)	• CP	6.16 y ($\bar{x}$) Required: ≥3 mo	91 pts received • 8 visits: • 12 wk (1x/wk for 4 wk; 1x/2 wk for 4 wk) 55 pts received • 30 h total over 6 d	• TPR	Additive techniques: • PRT Comparison groups: N/A	N/A	PPSS urinary: • Baseline: 9.6[c] • Post-tx: 5.7[c]	PPSS sexual total: • Baseline: 5.0[c] • Post-tx: 3.4[c] PPSS sexual: difficulty achieving erection: • Baseline: 70 subjects • Post-tx: 33/70 (47%)	PPSS pain: All subjects: • Baseline: 14.3[c] • Post-tx: 10.1[c] Subjects c/ ejaculatory pain: • Baseline: 81 people • Post-tx: 38/81 (47%)	Weak Evidence that: • <50% may have a ≥50% improvement in pain c/ejaculation (47%), and PPSS scores of: overall pain (39%), sexual fxn (43%), and urinary fxn (38%)

(continued on next page)

Table 2
(*continued*)

Author and Year	LOER, Study Type, PEDro Rating	Subject Characteristics: N, Sex	Age (y)	Medical Dx	Duration of Sx	Intervention Details: Frequency and Duration	Manual PT Techniques	Additional or Comparative Techniques	Results: Function: Bowel	Bladder	Sexual	Pain	Reviewers' Conclusions
											reported a ≥50% improvement PPSS sexual: difficulty maintaining erection: • Baseline: 64 subjects • Post-tx: 33/64 (52%) reported a ≥50% improvement PPSS sexual: difficulty achieving ejaculation: • Baseline: 64 subjects • Post-tx: 33/64 (52%) reported a ≥50% improvement	reported a ≥50% improvement NIH-CPSI pain: • Baseline: 11.5[c] • Post-tx: 8.5[c]	Other: • Likely a repeat population of the 2005 study • Looking several variables • <50% perceived a marked improvement in symptoms (GRA) • 2 different protocols administered—unable to discern which freq/duration most effective
Downey & Frederick,[67] 2005	4: Case study, pretest/posttest, 2/10	1, ♂: 0, ♀: 1	25	• Vulvar vestibulitis	3.25 y	• 8 visits	• Massage: (R) side of introitus, sweeping between 3- to 9-o'clock positions c/mod pressure	Additive techniques: • BF: contract/relax c/ emphasis on relaxation • HEP: PFM contraction	N/A	N/A	N/A	NPRS: Speculum insertion: • Baseline: 8.5/10 • 2-mo f/u: 0.5/10 Levatori ani palpation:	Weak Evidence that: • Manual techniques in addition to BF and HEP will significantly decrease pain with speculum insertion, pain

							• Stretching: 1 finger at 5- and 1 at 7-o'clock position of the introitus	3–10 s holds, 10 reps, 2x/d Comparison groups: N/A				• 4th visit: 2/10 on (R) side and 3/10 on (L) side • 7th visit: 2/10 • 8th visit: 0/10 • 2-mo f/u: 0/10	with palpation, & pt perspective of severity Other: • Pt uncomfortable performing self-massage at home • Pt's primary exercises were PFM contractions, focused on relaxation → hard to determine that the manual techniques lead to improvements • No definition of moderate pressure
Anderson et al,[60] 2005	4: Case series, retrospective, pretest/posttest, 2/10	138, ♂: 138, ♀: 0	40.5 ($\bar{x}$) (16–79)	• CP • Orchalgia	2.6 y (med)	• 5 visits (med) • 1x/wk for 4 wk followed by 1x/2 wk for 8 wk	• TPR: 60 s • Deep tissue mobilization (stripping, strumming, skin rolling and effleurage)	Additive techniques: • Ther ex: contract/relax of PFMs • PRT: 1 h/wk for 8 wk; pt instructed to continue relaxation sessions at home 1 h/d for 6 mo	N/A	PPSS urinary: • 37% of pts had ≥50% improvement in urinary symptoms	PPSS sexual: • 51% had ≥50% improvement in sexual fxn	PPSS pain: • 39% had ≥50% improvement in pain NPRS: • 36% had ≥50% improvement in pain	Weak Evidence that: • <40% of pts had ≥50% improvement in urinary sx and pain • Largest improvement in sexual fxn outcome measure: 51% of pts had a >50% improvement

(*continued on next page*)

Table 2
(continued)

Author and Year	LOER, Study Type, PEDro Rating	Subject Characteristics: N, Sex	Subject Characteristics: Age (y)	Subject Characteristics: Medical Dx	Subject Characteristics: Duration of Sx	Intervention Details: Frequency and Duration	Intervention Details: Manual PT Techniques	Intervention Details: Additional or Comparative Techniques	Results: Function: Bowel	Results: Function: Bladder	Results: Function: Sexual	Results: Pain	Reviewers' Conclusions
								Comparison groups: N/A					Other: • PPSS was not validated • Did not provide data tables with actual numbers, only % decrease • Assessing several variables • Authors included anything above 25% improvement as significant, reviewer has different definition of significant improvement
Oyama et al,[69] 2004	4: Case series, Prospective pilot study, 2/10	21, ♂: 0, ♀: 21	42 ($\bar{x}$) (21–64)	• IC	5–14 y	• 10 visits • 5 min • 2x/w for 5 wk	• Thiele massage: 10–15 reps from O to I • TPR: 10–15 s at pt's discretion	Additive techniques: N/A Comparison groups: N/A	N/A	ICPI: • Baseline: 8.2 • Post-tx: 6.3 • Long term: 5.1 ICSI: • Baseline: 8.9	N/A	Likert VAS for pain: • Baseline: 5.4 • Post-tx: 3.5 • Long-term 2.6	Weak Evidence for: • Significant improvement in ICPI, ICSI, and pain scores; maintained at 4.5-mo f/u

• Post-tx: 6.9 • Long-term: 5.1 Likert VAS for urgency: • Baseline: 4.6 • Post-tx: 3.0 • Long-term: 3.2	• Significant improvement in urgency symptoms, but were starting to decline f/u Other: • Did not maintain QoL gains • Only 62% at the long-term f/u assessment • Defined the pain scale as a Likert VAS; however, may be mislabeled • No tables provided for outcome measures

Definition of terms:

Manual physical therapy techniques: includes massage and trigger point release applied to the pelvic floor muscles and surrounding structures; for the purposes of this investigation joint mobilization and manipulation are not included.

Function: bowel, bladder, and sexual function, including but not limited to urinary continence/frequency/urgency/hesitancy, ability to defecate and ability to engage in sexual intercourse.

Patients: men or women; adults (≥18 years old).

Pelvic pain: pain in the pelvic region of men or women, which is nonmalignant in origin.[83]

Abbreviations: (B), bilateral; (L), left; (R), right; ($\bar{x}$), mean; ab, abdominal; c/, with; BF, biofeedback; CP, chronic prostatitis; CTM, connective tissue manipulation; ctrls, controls; DEC, decrease; e-stim, electrical stimulation; EGS, electrogalvanic stimulation; f/u, follow-up; Freq, frequency; FSFI 2000, female sexual functioning index; fxn, function; GTM, global therapeutic massage; HEP, home exercise program; IBS, irritable bowel syndrome; IC, interstitial cystitis; ICPI, O'Leary-Sant IC problem index; ICSI, O'Leary-Sant IC symptom index; INC, increase; LAS, levator ani syndrome; LE, lower extremity; LOER, level of evidence rating; Med, median; MHP, moist heat pack; mod, moderate; MPT, myofascial physical therapy; N/A, not applicable; NIH-CPSI, National Institutes of Health chronic prostatitis symptom index; NOS, not otherwise specified; NPRS, numeric pain rating scale; O to I, origin to insertion; PEDro; physiotherapy evidence database; PF(M), pelvic floor (muscles); proximal interphalengeal joint; PIP, proximal interphalengeal joint; PPSS, Pelvic Pain Symptom Survey; PRT, paradoxical relaxation training; Psych, psychologist; PT, physical therapy/physical therapist; pt(s), patient(s); PVD, provoked vestibulodynia; QoL, quality of life; RCT, randomized controlled trial; ROM, range of motion; SHIM, sexual health inventory for men; SS-SE, sexuality scale—sexual esteem subscale; SUI, stress urinary incontinence; Sx, symptoms; T10, 10th thoracic vertebra; TA, transverse abdominus; TP(s), trigger point(s); TPR, trigger point release; Tx, treatment; UE, upper extremity; UUI, urge urinary incontinence; VAS, visual analog scale; x, times.

[a] Numbers were estimated/averaged based on data provided in Tables 1 and 3 of the authors' article.

[b] Numbers were averaged based on data provided in Table 1 of the authors' article.

[c] Numbers were averaged based on data provided in Table 4 of the authors' article.

Data from Refs.[56–60,62–69,83]

SUMMARY

The cause of myofascial pain is currently unknown. Individuals with complaints of pain in the pelvic region should undergo a physical examination to determine the presence of pain with palpation of the muscles in the pelvic region. Conservative interventions should be considered to address the impairments found on physical examination.

REFERENCES

1. Apte G, Nelson P, Brismee JM, et al. Chronic female pelvic pain–part 1: clinical pathoanatomy and examination of the pelvic region. Pain Pract 2012;12(2): 88–110.
2. Grace VM, Zondervan KT. Chronic pelvic pain in New Zealand: prevalence, pain severity, diagnoses and use of the health services. Aust N Z J Public Health 2004;28(4):369–75.
3. Jarrell J. Endometriosis and abdominal myofascial pain in adults and adolescents. Curr Pain Headache Rep 2011;15(5):368–76.
4. Warren JW, Morozov V, Howard FM, et al. Before the onset of interstitial cystitis/bladder pain syndrome, the presence of multiple non-bladder syndromes is strongly associated with a history of multiple surgeries. J Psychosom Res 2014;76(1):75–9.
5. Paulson JD, Delgado M. Chronic pelvic pain: the occurrence of interstitial cystitis in a gynecological population. JSLS 2005;9(4):426–30.
6. Reiter RC. Evidence-based management of chronic pelvic pain. Clin Obstet Gynecol 1998;41(2):422–35.
7. Kotarinos R. Myofascial pelvic pain. Curr Pain Headache Rep 2012;16(5):433–8.
8. Wheeler AH. Myofascial pain disorders: theory to therapy. Drugs 2004;64(1): 45–62.
9. Newham AP, van der Spuy ZM, Nugent F. Laparoscopic findings in women with chronic pelvic pain. S Afr Med J 1996;86(9 Suppl):1200–3.
10. Howard FM. The role of laparoscopy in the chronic pelvic pain patient. Clin Obstet Gynecol 2003;46(4):749–66.
11. Skootsky SA, Jaeger B, Oye RK. Prevalence of myofascial pain in general internal medicine practice. West J Med 1989;151(2):157–60.
12. Bielefeldt K, Lamb K, Gebhart GF. Convergence of sensory pathways in the development of somatic and visceral hypersensitivity. Am J Physiol Gastrointest Liver Physiol 2006;291(4):G658–65.
13. Baskin LS, Tanagho EA. Pelvic pain without pelvic organs. J Urol 1992;147(3): 683–6.
14. Simons DG, Travell JG, Simmons LS. Myofascial pain and dysfunction: the trigger point manual. 2nd edition. Baltimore (MD): Williams and Wilkins; 1999.
15. Mense S. The pathogenesis of muscle pain. Curr Pain Headache Rep 2003;7(6): 419–25.
16. Kuner R. Central mechanisms of pathological pain. Nat Med 2010;16(11): 1258–66.
17. Sahrmann SA. The human movement system: our professional identity. Phys Ther 2014. [Epub ahead of print].
18. Sahrmann SA. Twenty-ninth Mary McMillan lecture: moving precisely? Or taking the path of least resistance? Phys Ther 1998;78:1208–18.
19. Sola AE, Rodenberger ML, Gettys BB. Incidence of hypersensitive areas in posterior shoulder muscles; a survey of two hundred young adults. Am J Phys Med 1955;34(6):585–90.

20. Gerwin RD, Dommerholt J, Shah JP. An expansion of Simons' integrated hypothesis of trigger point formation. Curr Pain Headache Rep 2004;8(6):468–75.
21. Shah JP, Gilliams EA. Uncovering the biochemical milieu of myofascial trigger points using in vivo microdialysis: an application of muscle pain concepts to myofascial pain syndrome. J Bodyw Mov Ther 2008;12(4):371–84.
22. Spitznagle TM. Musculoskeletal chronic pelvic pain. In: Carriere B, Feldt C, editors. Pelvic Floor. Stuttgart (Germany): Georg Thieme Verlag; 2006. p. 35–64.
23. Prather H, Spitznagle TM, Dugan SA. Recognizing and treating pelvic pain and pelvic floor dysfunction. Phys Med Rehabil Clin N Am 2007;18(3):477–96, ix.
24. Simons DG. New views of myofascial trigger points: etiology and diagnosis. Arch Phys Med Rehabil 2008;89(1):157–9.
25. Hyldahl RD, Hubal MJ. Lengthening our perspective: morphological, cellular, and molecular responses to eccentric exercise. Muscle Nerve 2014;49(2): 155–70.
26. Bron C, Dommerholt JD. Etiology of myofascial trigger points. Curr Pain Headache Rep 2012;16(5):439–44.
27. Meltzer KR, Cao TV, Schad JF, et al. In vitro modeling of repetitive motion injury and myofascial release. J Bodyw Mov Ther 2010;14(2):162–71.
28. Weiss JM. Pelvic floor myofascial trigger points: manual therapy for interstitial cystitis and the urgency-frequency syndrome. J Urol 2001;166(6):2226–31.
29. Spitznagle TM, Sahrmann S. Diagnosis and treatment of 2 adolescent female athletes with transient abdominal pain during running. J Sport Rehabil 2011; 20(2):228–49.
30. Van Dillen LR, Sahrmann SA, Norton BJ, et al. Effect of active limb movements on symptoms in patients with low back pain. J Orthop Sports Phys Ther 2001; 31(8):402–13.
31. Van Dillen LR, Sahrmann SA, Norton BJ, et al. The effect of modifying patient-preferred spinal movement and alignment during symptom testing in patients with low back pain: a preliminary report. Arch Phys Med Rehabil 2003;84(3): 313–22.
32. Harris-Hayes M, Van Dillen LR, Sahrmann SA. Classification, treatment and outcomes of a patient with lumbar extension syndrome. Physiother Theory Pract 2005;21(3):181–96.
33. Harris-Hayes M, Sahrmann SA, Norton BJ, et al. Diagnosis and management of a patient with knee pain using the movement system impairment classification system. J Orthop Sports Phys Ther 2008;38(4):203–13.
34. Van Dillen LR, McDonnell MK, Susco TM, et al. The immediate effect of passive scapular elevation on symptoms with active neck rotation in patients with neck pain. Clin J Pain 2007;23(8):641–7.
35. McDonnell MK, Sahrmann SA, Van DL. A specific exercise program and modification of postural alignment for treatment of cervicogenic headache: a case report. J Orthop Sports Phys Ther 2005;35(1):3–15.
36. Caldwell C, Sahrmann S, Van DL. Use of a movement system impairment diagnosis for physical therapy in the management of a patient with shoulder pain. J Orthop Sports Phys Ther 2007;37(9):551–63.
37. Burkholder TJ, Fingado B, Baron S, et al. Relationship between muscle fiber types and sizes and muscle architectural properties in the mouse hindlimb. J Morphol 1994;221(2):177–90.
38. Tuttle LJ, Nguyen OT, Cook MS, et al. Architectural design of the pelvic floor is consistent with muscle functional subspecialization. Int Urogynecol J 2014; 25(2):205–12.

39. Gerwin RD, Shannon S, Hong CZ, et al. Interrater reliability in myofascial trigger point examination. Pain 1997;69(1–2):65–73.
40. Hsieh CY, Hong CZ, Adams AH, et al. Interexaminer reliability of the palpation of trigger points in the trunk and lower limb muscles. Arch Phys Med Rehabil 2000; 81(3):258–64.
41. Nice DA, Riddle DL, Lamb RL, et al. Intertester reliability of judgments of the presence of trigger points in patients with low back pain. Arch Phys Med Rehabil 1992;73(10):893–8.
42. Njoo KH, Van der DE. The occurrence and inter-rater reliability of myofascial trigger points in the quadratus lumborum and gluteus medius: a prospective study in non-specific low back pain patients and controls in general practice. Pain 1994;58(3):317–23.
43. Wolfe F, Simons DG, Fricton J, et al. The fibromyalgia and myofascial pain syndromes: a preliminary study of tender points and trigger points in persons with fibromyalgia, myofascial pain syndrome and no disease. J Rheumatol 1992; 19(6):944–51.
44. Reeves JL, Jaeger B, Graff-Radford SB. Reliability of the pressure algometer as a measure of myofascial trigger point sensitivity. Pain 1986;24(3):313–21.
45. Tu FF, Fitzgerald CM, Kuiken T, et al. Comparative measurement of pelvic floor pain sensitivity in chronic pelvic pain. Obstet Gynecol 2007;110(6):1244–8.
46. Tu FF, Fitzgerald CM, Kuiken T, et al. Vaginal pressure-pain thresholds: initial validation and reliability assessment in healthy women. Clin J Pain 2008;24(1):45–50.
47. Shah JP, Phillips TM, Danoff JV, et al. An in vivo microanalytical technique for measuring the local biochemical milieu of human skeletal muscle. J Appl Physiol (1985) 2005;99(5):1977–84.
48. Chen Q, Bensamoun S, Basford JR, et al. Identification and quantification of myofascial taut bands with magnetic resonance elastography. Arch Phys Med Rehabil 2007;88(12):1658–61.
49. Ballyns JJ, Shah JP, Hammond J, et al. Objective sonographic measures for characterizing myofascial trigger points associated with cervical pain. J Ultrasound Med 2011;30(10):1331–40.
50. Sikdar S, Ortiz R, Gebreab T, et al. Understanding the vascular environment of myofascial trigger points using ultrasonic imaging and computational modeling. Conf Proc IEEE Eng Med Biol Soc 2010;2010:5302–5.
51. Sikdar S, Shah JP, Gebreab T, et al. Novel applications of ultrasound technology to visualize and characterize myofascial trigger points and surrounding soft tissue. Arch Phys Med Rehabil 2009;90(11):1829–38.
52. Sikdar S, Shah JP, Gilliams E, et al. Assessment of myofascial trigger points (MTrPs): a new application of ultrasound imaging and vibration sonoelastography. Conf Proc IEEE Eng Med Biol Soc 2008;2008:5585–8.
53. Turo D, Otto P, Shah JP, et al. Ultrasonic characterization of the upper trapezius muscle in patients with chronic neck pain. Ultrason Imaging 2013;35(2):173–87.
54. Maher RM, Hayes DM, Shinohara M. Quantification of dry needling and posture effects on myofascial trigger points using ultrasound shear-wave elastography. Arch Phys Med Rehabil 2013;94(11):2146–50.
55. Fitzgerald MP, Anderson RU, Potts J, et al. Randomized multicenter feasibility trial of myofascial physical therapy for the treatment of urological chronic pelvic pain syndromes. J Urol 2013;189(Suppl 1):S75–85.
56. Fitzgerald MP, Payne CK, Lukacz ES, et al. Randomized multicenter clinical trial of myofascial physical therapy in women with interstitial cystitis/painful bladder syndrome and pelvic floor tenderness. J Urol 2012;187(6):2113–8.

57. Fitzgerald MP, Anderson RU, Potts J, et al. Randomized multicenter feasibility trial of myofascial physical therapy for the treatment of urological chronic pelvic pain syndromes. J Urol 2009;182(2):570–80.
58. Van Alstyne LS, Harrington KL, Haskvitz EM. Physical therapist management of chronic prostatitis/chronic pelvic pain syndrome. Phys Ther 2010;90(12): 1795–806.
59. Chiarioni G, Nardo A, Vantini I, et al. Biofeedback is superior to electrogalvanic stimulation and massage for treatment of levator ani syndrome. Gastroenterology 2010;138(4):1321–9.
60. Anderson RU, Wise D, Sawyer T, et al. Integration of myofascial trigger point release and paradoxical relaxation training treatment of chronic pelvic pain in men. J Urol 2005;174(1):155–60.
61. Anderson RU. Traditional therapy for chronic pelvic pain does not work: what do we do now? Nat Clin Pract Urol 2006;3(3):145–56.
62. Anderson RU, Wise D, Sawyer T, et al. 6-day intensive treatment protocol for refractory chronic prostatitis/chronic pelvic pain syndrome using myofascial release and paradoxical relaxation training. J Urol 2011;185(4):1294–9.
63. Gentilcore-Saulnier E, McLean L, Goldfinger C, et al. Pelvic floor muscle assessment outcomes in women with and without provoked vestibulodynia and the impact of a physical therapy program. J Sex Med 2010;7(2 Pt 2): 1003–22.
64. Goldfinger C, Pukall CF, Gentilcore-Saulnier E, et al. A prospective study of pelvic floor physical therapy: pain and psychosexual outcomes in provoked vestibulodynia. J Sex Med 2009;6(7):1955–68.
65. Olszewski RM. Case report of a postpartum patient with vestibulodynia, dyspareunia, constipatoni and stress urinary incontinence. J Womens Health Phys Therap 2012;36(1):20–34.
66. Figures CC, Amundsen CL, Weidner AC, et al. Physical therapy intervensions for voiding dysfunction and pelvic pain; a retrospective case series. J Womens Health Phys Therap 2010;34(2):40–4.
67. Downey PA, Frederick I. Physical therapy treatment for vulvar vestibulitis: a case report. J Womens Health Phys Therap 2005;29(3):16–9.
68. Anderson RU, Wise D, Sawyer T, et al. Sexual dysfunction in men with chronic prostatitis/chronic pelvic pain syndrome: improvement after trigger point release and paradoxical relaxation training. J Urol 2006;176(4 Pt 1):1534–8.
69. Oyama IA, Rejba A, Lukban JC, et al. Modified Thiele massage as therapeutic intervention for female patients with interstitial cystitis and high-tone pelvic floor dysfunction. Urology 2004;64(5):862–5.
70. Singh S, Nagaraj C, Khare GN, et al. Multicentric tuberculosis at two rare sites in an immunocompetent adult. J Orthop Traumatol 2011;12(4):223–5.
71. Arendt-Nielsen L, Schipper KP, Dimcevski G, et al. Viscero-somatic reflexes in referred pain areas evoked by capsaicin stimulation of the human gut. Eur J Pain 2008;12(5):544–51.
72. Chun AA, McGee SR. Bedside diagnosis of coronary artery disease: a systematic review. Am J Med 2004;117(5):334–43.
73. Jarrell J. Gynecological pain, endometriosis, visceral disease and the Viscerosomatic connection. J Muscskel Health 2008;16:21–7.
74. Stawowy M, Bluhme C, Arendt-Nielsen L, et al. Somatosensory changes in the referred pain area in patients with acute cholecystitis before and after treatment with laparoscopic or open cholecystectomy. Scand J Gastroenterol 2004; 39(10):988–93.

75. Giamberardino MA, Affaitati G, Lerza R, et al. Relationship between pain symptoms and referred sensory and trophic changes in patients with gallbladder pathology. Pain 2005;114(1–2):239–49.
76. Giamberardino MA, Costantini R, Affaitati G, et al. Viscero-visceral hyperalgesia: characterization in different clinical models. Pain 2010;151(2):307–22.
77. Bevilaqua-Grossi D, Lipton RB, Napchan U, et al. Temporomandibular disorders and cutaneous allodynia are associated in individuals with migraine. Cephalalgia 2010;30(4):425–32.
78. Janig W, Habler HJ. Physiology and pathophysiology of visceral pain. Schmerz 2002;16(6):429–46 [in German].
79. Rose WD, Veach JS, Tehranzdeh J. Spontaneous pneumomediastinum as a cause of neck pain, dysphagia, and chest pain. Arch Intern Med 1984;144(2):392–3.
80. McGee TC, Field RS, Loebl DH, et al. Pustulotic arthro-osteitis: a cause of atypical chest pain and a new arthritic syndrome. South Med J 1993;86(4):469–72.
81. Drapanas T, Yates AJ, Brickman R, et al. The syndrome of occult rupture of the spleen. Arch Surg 1969;99(3):298–306.
82. Giamberardino MA, de Bigontina P, Martegiani C, et al. Effects of extracorporeal shock-wave lithotripsy on referred hyperalgesia from renal/ureteral calculosis. Pain 1994;56(1):77–83.
83. Messelink B, Benson T, Berghmans B, et al. Standardization of terminology of pelvic floor muscle function and dysfunction: report from the pelvic floor clinical assessment group of the international continence society. Neurourol Urodyn 2005;24:374–80.

Musculoskeletal Etiologies of Pelvic Pain

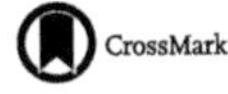

Heidi Prather, DO[a,*], Alejandra Camacho-Soto, MD[b]

KEYWORDS

• Musculoskeletal • Lumbar spine • Pelvic pain • Pelvic girdle

KEY POINTS

- Pelvic pain includes disorders of the musculoskeletal system.
- Visceral disorders of the pelvis can be associated with musculoskeletal pelvic pain and dysfunction.
- Musculoskeletal disorders associated with pelvic pain may develop from disorders of the lumbar spine, pelvic girdle and hip.
- It is important for clinicians to assess for more than a single structure as a source of pelvic pain.

MUSCULOSKELETAL DIAGNOSES OUTSIDE OF THE PELVIC GIRDLE

Nature of the Problem

An estimated 22% of musculoskeletal diagnoses are frequently concomitant with pelvic floor pathology and pain.[1] The definition of pelvic pain itself often depends on the medical specialist evaluating the patient. To a urologist, this may be defined as a visceral disorder associated with visceral and somatic pain of the pelvic floor. A physiatrist may consider a pelvic girdle somatic disorder and its relationship to the hip and spine as sources of pain. Because there is such variability among disorders associated with pelvic pain, patients may seek treatment for extended periods as various treatment options are attempted. Further, health care providers should recognize that there may not be a single source of dysfunction. Patients with a painful bladder often have compensatory elevated resting pelvic floor muscle tone that results in concomitant muscle pain. Patients with S1 radiculopathy may develop increased resting tone of pelvic floor as compensation that leads to pelvic floor

No financial disclosures.

[a] Section of Physical Medicine and Rehabilitation, Department of Orthopaedic Surgery, Washington University School of Medicine, 660 South Euclid Avenue, Campus Box 8233, St Louis, MO 63110, USA; [b] Department of Physical Medicine and Rehabilitation, Northwestern University Feinberg School of Medicine/Rehabilitation Institute of Chicago, 345 East Superior Street, Chicago, IL 60611, USA

* Corresponding author.

E-mail address: pratherh@wustl.edu

Obstet Gynecol Clin N Am 41 (2014) 433–442
http://dx.doi.org/10.1016/j.ogc.2014.04.004 obgyn.theclinics.com
0889-8545/14/$ – see front matter

muscle pain. An increase in low back pain (LBP) may then be related to the increased intradiscal pressure created by increased pelvic pressure. The problem becomes cyclical, and the health care provider is challenged with what to offer to best break the cycle.

This article discusses the musculoskeletal disorders of the pelvic girdle (structures within the bony pelvis) and their association with lumbar spine and hip disorders.

It is essential for health care providers to consider these musculoskeletal diagnoses when evaluating patients with pelvic pain. Although musculoskeletal pathology may not be the primary cause, screening for and treating potential contributors to pelvic pain may lead to better treatment plans and avoidance of unnecessary procedures. Given the large percentage of patients with chronic pelvic pain of unknown cause undergoing surgical procedures, the American College of Obstetrics and Gynecology recommends a musculoskeletal evaluation before laparoscopy or hysterectomy. Because there is an overlap in disorders resulting in pelvic girdle pain (PGP), definitions for these musculoskeletal disorders in isolation are provided here.[2]

Definition

Pelvic girdle pain as defined by European guidelines for pelvic girdle pain

PGP generally arises in relation to pregnancy, trauma, arthritis, and osteoarthritis. Pain is experienced between the posterior iliac crest and the gluteal fold, particularly in the vicinity of the sacroiliac joint (SIJ). The pain may radiate in the posterior thigh and can also occur in conjunction with, or separately in, the symphysis. The endurance capacity for standing, walking, and sitting is diminished. The diagnosis of PGP is reached after exclusion of lumbar causes. The pain or functional disturbances in relation to PGP must be reproducible by specific clinical tests.

SPINE

Nature of the Problem

The lumbosacral roots, plexus, and peripheral nerves innervate the pelvic floor; therefore, pathology affecting the lumbar spine may present with overlapping symptoms due to the distribution of innervation and referral patterns. Lumbar spine disorders may refer pain in the distribution of the groin, with or without associated LBP. Lumbosacral plexopathies can occur secondary to trauma, tumor, metastatic lesions, and radiation-induced treatment effects.

Definitions

Discogenic pain: pain attributed to the intervertebral disc without radiating pain or sensory symptoms into the lower extremities.

Radicular pain: pain that radiates into the lower extremities within the distribution of the nerve root affected with no associated neurologic deficits.

Radiculopathy: sensory and/or motor deficits in a nerve root distribution with or without pain as a result of nerve root compression.

Lumbar plexopathy: pain that radiates to the lower extremities distal to the nerve root, from the lumbosacral plexus (L1-S4), with further subdivisions of the plexus.

Symptom Criteria

Patients may complain of LBP and buttock, thigh, groin, pelvis, or leg pain. Pain associated with radiculopathies and plexopathies often radiate into the pelvis or lower extremities in a dermatomal distribution. Sacral radiculopathies (S2-S4) may present with sensory deficits in the perineum and perianal areas, with possible bowel or bladder incontinence and sexual dysfunction. Screening for red flags such as progressive weakness, fevers, night sweats, unexplained weight loss, bowel or bladder incontinence, saddle anesthesia, and sexual dysfunction should prompt a more aggressive management and treatment plan.

Clinical findings

Patients commonly present with pain in the lumbar spine, pelvis, and lower extremity. It is important to assess for associated neurologic impairment such as progressive numbness or tingling in the lower extremity or weakness. Urgent evaluation of the lumbar spine with imaging should be performed if the patient presents with saddle anesthesia, progressive motor weakness, and bowel or bladder incontinence.

Physical Examination

When analyzing musculoskeletal disorders of the spine-hip-pelvis complex, the following tests should be included in all evaluations: gait analysis, range of motion, muscle strength testing of the lower extremities, deep tendon reflexes, and sensation, noting any asymmetry between sides. Special tests function as potential screening or confirmatory tests. The special tests straight leg raise, crossed straight leg raise, and slump test have shown a sensitivity and specificity of 0.92 for nerve root compression in lumbosacral spine disorders.[3]

Diagnostic Modalities

Electrodiagnostic studies may help identify the level of injury and distinguish between radiculopathies and plexopathies in patients with focal weakness or sensory impairments. Selective nerve root blocks have been used as both diagnostic and treatment modalities for radicular pain, although a recent review showed limited evidence for its use as a diagnostic tool for LBP with radicular symptoms.[4]

Imaging

According to Jarvik and Deyo,[5] imaging can be deferred in uncomplicated back pain if the patient is less than 50 years old with no identified red flags, no history of cancer, and no neurologic deficits on examination. The most common imaging tests ordered to assess for spine structural disorders are anteroposterior and lateral plain radiographs, which illustrate the bony architecture and alignment. Computed tomographic (CT) scans have similar sensitivity and specificity compared with magnetic resonance imaging (MRI) for identifying herniated discs. If history and examination reveal any red flags, the patient should have an MRI of their lumbosacral spine with and without contrast to evaluate for metastatic disease, infection, and nerve root compression, which may require urgent surgical intervention. An MRI of the pelvis is the most sensitive of imaging modalities in differentiating between radiation-induced injury and tumor in lumbosacral plexopathies.[6]

Pathology

Normal aging is associated with degeneration of intervertebral discs, spondylosis (arthritic changes in the spine), and loss of bone density, all conditions that may predispose patients to pathologic changes subsequently resulting in pain. Radicular pain associated with a lumbosacral radiculopathy may be secondary to a herniated disc, central or foraminal stenosis that may or may not be associated with nerve root compression. The structural sources for axial LBP are not fully understood and commonly a source of debate among spine specialists. There continues to be an increasing body of literature that suggests subgrouping of patients with specific characteristics and whose symptoms increase and improve with specific movement patterns. This type of diagnostic grouping allows for greater diagnostic specificity, which leads to a more specific directed treatment.

Diagnostic Dilemmas

Process of elimination

Distinguishing the potential cause of the pain from the level of the anterior horn cell of the spinal cord to the peripheral nerve is challenging but should always start with a thorough history and examination. Upper motor neuron findings such as increased reflexes suggest central nervous system disorders, whereas lower motor neuron findings such as reduced reflexes suggest a peripheral nervous system disorder. Motor neuron disorders can have mixed upper and lower motor neuron changes. Although there are limitations to imaging and electrodiagnostic testing, a combination of findings can help support a diagnosis in the lumbar spine.

Summary

There is overlap in symptoms of women with PGP and the lumbar spine disorder. A lumbar spine disorder is best assessed with an appropriate history and physical examination. When neurologic symptoms are present or if the patient fails to improve with treatment, an MRI of the lumbar spine is indicated. Not all findings indicate a source of pain. The patient symptom complex should be assessed with the findings to better determine the diagnosis and course of treatment.

HIP

Nature of the Problem

Pain related to a hip disorder can present with a wide distribution of pain, including posterior pelvis, groin, circumferential thigh and calf pain.[7] Because muscles that provide stability and allow motion of the hip are located in the pelvic floor, patients may also present with pelvic floor pain. The causes of hip pain are divided into intra-articular and extra-articular diagnoses, with the following intra-articular pathologies discussed later.

Definitions

Hip osteoarthritis: degeneration of the cartilage in the hip joint resulting in loss of protective forces, resulting in pain.

Hip acetabular labral tear: tear of the ring of fibrocartilage in the hip joint, which surrounds the acetabulum (with the exception of the inferior surface).

Femoroacetabular impingement: this definition contains 5 essential elements: (1) abnormal morphology of the femur and/or acetabulum, (2) abnormal contact between these 2 structures, (3) motion that results in abnormal contact, (4) repetitive motion resulting in the continuous insult, and (5) the presence of soft-tissue damage. This set of circumstances promotes cartilage injury leading to osteoarthritis.[8]

Congenital and developmental hip dysplasia: hip dysplasia includes a group of disorders that have deformities of the joint characterized by a shallow socket that does not adequately cover the femoral head. When the femoral head is not completely covered by the acetabulum, the hip is unstable, may become painful, and may eventually develop osteoarthritis.

Hip stress fracture: a break in the bone that occurs when minor injuries to the bone build up beyond the capacity of the bone to repair itself.

Hip osteonecrosis: vascular compromise to the bone, most commonly affecting the femoral head, which leads to cell death and collapse.

Symptom Criteria

Symptoms of osteoarthritis may include morning stiffness and pain with weight bearing activities, with progression of pain at rest as the disease progresses. Acetabular labral tears can occur in isolation but are more commonly associated with hip deformity (developmental hip dysplasia [DDH] and femoroacetabular impingement [FAI]). Symptoms associated with this group of disorders include insidious onset and pain described as sharp and/or dull with mechanical symptoms such as locking, catching, or giving way.[9] Activities that may exacerbate symptoms include hip extension, prolonged walking and sitting, and pivoting. Unique to patients with FAI is the common finding of reduced hip flexion and internal passive range of motion. Hip stress fractures may present as exercise-induced pain during weight bearing, with almost complete resolution with rest.

Clinical Findings

Physical examination

There is a combination of physical examination tests used to support a diagnosis of hip pathology. These include the anterior hip impingement test (90° in hip flexion, adduction, and internal rotation), FABER or Patrick test (hip *f*lexion, *ab*duction, and *e*xternal *r*otation), and the resisted straight leg test (supine with leg raised to 45° with resistance from clinician).[10] In osteoarthritis, hip range of motion is restricted first in internal rotation and can progress to involve all planes of motion. A Trendelenburg gait on examination is common in hip pathology, secondary to a weak gluteus medius, a muscle involved in hip abduction and internal rotation.

Diagnostic modalities

Diagnostic intra-articular hip injections with image guidance have a high sensitivity for assessment of intra-articular pain.[11]

Imaging

If a hip disorder is suspected, radiographs should be obtained to evaluate for bone abnormalities and alignment. Radiographs alone can describe osteoarthritis, fracture, stress fractures, deformity, and avascular necrosis. If radiographs are normal or show mild deformity, the next step is a diagnostic (anesthetic only) image-guided intra-articular injection. After injection, if the patient reports reduction in pain, a magnetic resonance (MR) arthrogram is the next step to diagnosing an intra-articular hip disorder. MR arthrography of the hip is the most sensitive (0.90) and specific (0.91) imaging modality for diagnosing labral tears.[12] For patients with contraindications to MR arthrography, a CT with contrast can be ordered with similar sensitivity and specificity.

Pathology

Osteoarthritis is associated with destruction and ongoing loss of articular cartilage with reactive bone changes resulting in hypertrophy and capsular thickening (osteophytes and spur formation at margins, subchondral sclerosis, and subchondral cyst formation.) In FAI, abnormal contact between the proximal femur and acetabulum may result in the development of labral tears and may increase the risk of developing osteoarthritis. DDH, most commonly diagnosed in infancy to early years, results in abnormal stresses within the joint, ongoing damage and development of osteoarthritis, and increased risk of labral tears. The labrum is a ringlike cartilaginous structure with layers of type 1 cartilage and hyaline cartilage that have many functions in the hip joint, including stabilization, preventing dislocation of the femoral head, deepening of the socket, and acting as a shock absorber. The thinnest portion of the labrum is found anteriorly, which is most susceptible to injury. The labrum has poor blood supply, supplying only the outer one-third of its external surface, yet a vast nerve supply with increased density in the anterior superior quadrant, resulting in pain if damaged.

Diagnostic dilemmas

Process of elimination Based on the American College of Rheumatology, hip osteoarthritis can be diagnosed with hip pain and 2 or more of the following: radiographic evidence of osteophytes, joint space narrowing, and an ESR less than 20. Hip osteoarthritis most commonly occurs in older adults. Two of the most common risk factors for osteonecrosis of the femoral head are corticosteroid use and alcohol abuse, representing 80% of cases. Risk factors associated with the development of stress fractures include female gender, amenorrhea, smoking, corticosteroid use, and the female triad. The female triad represents low energy availability or disordered eating, bone loss, and menstrual disturbances.

PUBIC DISORDERS

Nature of the Problem

The abdominal muscles, which provide core stability, insert into the pubic symphysis and surrounding bony structures. Consequently, abdominal muscle pathologic conditions, such as muscle tears or avulsions, frequently refer to the pelvis or groin area. Bony articular changes across the pubic symphysis related to trauma or chronic muscle imbalances can progress from acute inflammation (pubic symphysitis) to degenerative changes (osteitis pubis).

Definitions

Athletic pubalgia sports hernia: chronic groin pain from activity-related injury to the abdominal wall musculature attaching to or around the pubic symphysis.[13]

Pubic symphysitis: inflammation of the pubic symphysis.

Osteitis pubis: osteosclerosis of the pubic bone next to the symphysis, caused by trauma to that region.

Symptom Criteria

Symptoms are often insidious in onset, with unilateral groin pain radiating into the perineum and upper thigh.[14] Pain is worse with intense activity, and eventually affects less exertional activities such as coughing, sneezing, or moving in bed at night.[15] Pubic symphysitis may also present with pain with hip motion, especially adduction and abduction.

Clinical Findings

Physical examination

On palpation of the inguinal region, pubic tubercle, or along the muscle insertion during resisted sit-ups, the patient may complain of pain or tenderness. The Valsalva maneuver and resistance testing of hip adductors may reproduce the symptoms.[16] In addition, examination may reveal weakness in the lower abdominal muscles and reduced hip range of motion.[14] Pain on direct palpation of the pubic symphysis may indicate a joint or bony problem.

Diagnostic modalities

Imaging Radiographs of the pelvis assess bony abnormalities such as arthritis and fracture. Ultrasonography has been used as a diagnostic modality for dynamically visualizing tendon, muscle, and aponeurosis. It may reveal a tear, tendinopathy, or fluid collections.

A noncontrast MRI may reveal core muscle injury with a sensitivity and specificity of 68% and 100% for rectus abdominis injury and 86% and 89% for adductor tendon injury.[17]

Pathology

Diagnostic dilemmas

Process of elimination A diagnosis of sports hernia and pubic symphysitis is usually made on history taking and physical examination, using imaging to exclude other conditions. Athletic pubalgia is more common in sports with frequent sprinting, twisting, and turning. These symptoms usually resolve completely with cessation of activity. Pubic symphysitis and osteitis pubis may have the same presentation. Pubic symphysitis represents early intra-articular inflammation, whereas osteitis pubis represents an overload to bony structures, and when active, bone edema is noted on MRI. Direct palpation of the pubic region with reproduction of symptoms is commonly found in these disorders and not found in hip and spine disorders.

SACROILIAC JOINT PAIN

Nature of the Problem

Pain in the posterior pelvis is often labeled as SIJ pain based on location. In reality, pain in the posterior pelvis can be related to intra-articular SIJ, SIJ ligaments, and muscles of the pelvic. Because their mechanisms of action and therefore dysfunction overlap, likely these structures may not be painful in isolation. This theory would correlate with findings that there is no one objective test that rules in the diagnosis and that clusters of physical examination tests are needed to be positive to consider ruling in the diagnosis. Further, confirmation of the diagnosis often involves treatment such as an image-guided injection. SIJ pain may be considered in the diagnosis of LBP. This disorder has received the most attention from the lumbar spine community without a lot of consideration to what it implies at the pelvic girdle. For these reasons, adopting the term posterior pelvic girdle pain as discussed and reviewed by the authors of the European guidelines[2] instead of SIJ pain would be more representative of the potential dysfunctional and painful issues these patients experience.

Definitions

SIJ pain: pain in the region of the SIJ provoked by stressing the joint and relieved with injection.[18–20]

Posterior PGP: PGP generally arises in relation to pregnancy, trauma, arthritis, and osteoarthritis. Pain is experienced between the posterior iliac crest and the gluteal fold, particularly in the vicinity of the SIJ. The pain may radiate in the posterior thigh and can also occur in conjunction with, or separately in, the symphysis. The endurance capacity for standing, walking, and sitting is diminished. The diagnosis of PGP is reached after exclusion of lumbar causes. The pain or functional disturbances in relation to PGP must be reproducible by specific clinical tests.[2]

Symptom Criteria

Given the extensive innervation of the SIJ, symptoms frequently vary with complaints of pain in the low back below L5, into the buttock, groin, or leg. These symptoms may be exacerbated by prolonged positions such as sitting, standing, or lying supine. Pain may begin unilateral but can become bilateral. LBP referring into the groin may be more common in SIJ dysfunction than lumbar spine pathology alone.[21] Radiating symptoms past the knee is less common in patients with SIJ dysfunction but can occur.

Physical Examination

Provocative physical examination maneuvers that stress the SIJ include: distraction, FABER, sacral compression, Gaenslen, and sacral thrust. The tests are helpful in making a diagnosis of SIJ pain when clusters of these tests are positive but not when used in isolation.[22,23] The distraction test includes the application of lateral pressure over the iliac crests by the examiner with the patient in the supine position. The FABER test is performed with the patient in the supine position, and the examiner passively flexes and abducts the hip. The compression test is performed with the patient in the prone position, and compression is applied by the examiner across the sacral base. The Gaenslen test is performed with the patient in the supine position, with the ipsilateral leg dropped off the side of the table into hip extension while the opposite ilium is stabilized by the examiner. A test result is considered positive for any of these when the patient's posterior pelvic pain is reproduced. Often, greater than 50% pain relief with an image-guided intra-articular injection is considered the best mechanism to identify pain related to the SIJ.

Diagnostic Modalities

Pain relief after image-guided intra-articular injection of the SIJ with anesthetic is highly suggestive of SIJ dysfunction.

Imaging

Radiographic studies alone cannot diagnose SIJ pain and frequently are unremarkable for patient without inflammatory arthritis or spondyloarthropathies. Plain radiographs, CT, and MRI are used to rule out other potential causes of pain including: fracture, infection, tumor, and inflammatory arthritis.

PELVIC FLOOR

Nature of the Problem

Many patients with chronic pelvic pain have either increased or decreased resting tone of pelvic floor muscles. Similar to conditions outside of the pelvic girdle, muscles in the pelvic floor may present with trigger points or tenderness. Vaginal delivery and use of forceps in delivery are risk factors for decreased muscle strength in the pelvic floor for several years after childbirth. The muscles of the pelvic floor more commonly associated with pain symptoms include the coccygeus, levator ani, obturator internus, and piriformis, all of which are innervated by the sacral plexus.[24] These muscles assist in maintaining bowel and bladder continence, sexual function, and postural support. Increased tone is associated with shortening of the muscle fiber and eventual development of a contracture. Decreased muscle tone, fasciculations, and atrophy indicate muscle weakness.

Definitions

Pelvic floor muscle pain: persistent or recurrent, episodic, pelvic floor pain with associated trigger points, syndrome that is either related to the micturition cycle or associated with symptoms suggestive of urinary tract, bowel, or sexual dysfunction. No proven infection or other obvious pathology.[25]

Symptom Criteria

Symptoms described with pelvic floor dysfunction include dyspareunia, LBP, bowel or bladder incontinence, constipation, diarrhea, excessive flatus, painful defecation, urinary frequency, or urgency.[1] Pain and/or trigger points are commonly elicited on palpation of muscles and ligaments of the pelvic floor. Patient descriptions of quality of pain vary from aching, spasm, and burning. Commonly, patients may have visceral disorders such as painful bladder, endometriosis, or irritable bowel. There is increase in pelvic floor muscle tone, and ultimately, pain may develop in this setting.

Clinical Findings

Physical examination

Verbal consent should be obtained before performing the pelvic examination. A thorough inspection comparing sides for asymmetry such as atrophy, hypertrophy, or muscle spasms is indicated. A clock is commonly used for orientation to the anatomy and palpation, with the pubic bone at 12-o'clock position and the anus at 6-o'clock position. Tone is measured by visualizing the lift and descent of the perineal body and palpating the areas when the patient is asked to contract and relax the pelvic floor muscles. A Valsalva maneuver should be performed by the patient while observing the pelvic floor for bulging. Reflex testing is done by lightly moving a cotton tip applicator across the perineum and observing for the anal wink. The internal examination should assess for pain, tenderness, or increased tone, none of which should be positive without pathology. Similar to muscle outside of the pelvic girdle, trigger points should demonstrate increased tone and pain.

Diagnostic modalities

Increased muscle activity or a trigger point within the muscle is measured using electromyography. Diagnostic ultrasonography is used to assess the resting tone and ability to contract and relax the pelvic floor.

Imaging Imaging is used for ruling out other causes of pelvic pain such as tumors, infection, or diagnoses outside of the pelvic girdle.

Pathology

Commonly, pelvic floor muscle pain is associated with a musculoskeletal disorder related to the pelvic girdle, spine, or hip. Assessing these regions is imperative to treat the pelvic floor. Visceral disorders of the pelvic floor, such as painful bladder, endometriosis, and irritable bowel syndrome, may be associated with increased resting pelvic floor tone and pain.

REFERENCES

1. Gyang A, Hartman M, Lamvu G. Musculoskeletal causes of chronic pelvic pain: what a gynecologist should know. Obstet Gynecol 2013;121(3):645–50.
2. Vleeming A, Albert HB, Ostgaard HC, et al. European guidelines for the diagnosis and treatment of pelvic girdle pain. Eur Spine J 2008;17(6):794–819.
3. van der Windt DA, Simons E, Riphagen II, et al. Physical examination for lumbar radiculopathy due to disc herniation in patients with low-back pain. Cochrane Database Syst Rev 2010;(2):CD007431.
4. Datta S, Manchikanti L, Falco FJ, et al. Diagnostic utility of selective nerve root blocks in the diagnosis of lumbosacral radicular pain: systematic review and update of current evidence. Pain Physician 2013;16(Suppl 2):SE97–124.

5. Jarvik JG, Deyo RA. Diagnostic evaluation of low back pain with emphasis on imaging. Ann Intern Med 2002;137(7):586–97.
6. Taylor BV, Kimmel DW, Krecke KN, et al. Magnetic resonance imaging in cancer-related lumbosacral plexopathy. Mayo Clin Proc 1997;72(9):823–9.
7. Lesher JM, Dreyfuss P, Hager N, et al. Hip joint pain referral patterns: a descriptive study. Pain Med 2008;9(1):22–5.
8. Sankar WN, Nevitt M, Parvizi J, et al. Femoroacetabular impingement: defining the condition and its role in the pathophysiology of osteoarthritis. J Am Acad Orthop Surg 2013;21(Suppl 1):S7–15.
9. Burnett RS, Della Rocca GJ, Prather H, et al. Clinical presentation of patients with tears of the acetabular labrum. J Bone Joint Surg Am 2006;88(7):1448–57.
10. Tijssen M, van Cingel R, Willemsen L, et al. Diagnostics of femoroacetabular impingement and labral pathology of the hip: a systematic review of the accuracy and validity of physical tests. Arthroscopy 2012;28(6):860–71.
11. Byrd JW, Jones KS. Diagnostic accuracy of clinical assessment, magnetic resonance imaging, magnetic resonance arthrography, and intra-articular injection in hip arthroscopy patients. Am J Sports Med 2004;32(7):1668–74.
12. Genovese E, Spiga S, Vinci V, et al. Femoroacetabular impingement: role of imaging. Musculoskelet Surg 2013;97(Suppl 2):S117–26.
13. Brandon CJ, Jacobson JA, Fessell D, et al. Groin pain beyond the hip: how anatomy predisposes to injury as visualized by musculoskeletal ultrasound and MRI. AJR Am J Roentgenol 2011;197(5):1190–7.
14. Caudill P, Nyland J, Smith C, et al. Sports hernias: a systematic literature review. Br J Sports Med 2008;42(12):954–64.
15. Meyers WC, Kahan DM, Joseph T, et al. Current analysis of women athletes with pelvic pain. Med Sci Sports Exerc 2011;43(8):1387–93.
16. Taylor DC, Meyers WC, Moylan JA, et al. Abdominal musculature abnormalities as a cause of groin pain in athletes. Inguinal hernias and pubalgia. Am J Sports Med 1991;19(3):239–42.
17. Zoga AC, Kavanagh EC, Omar IM, et al. Athletic pubalgia and the "sports hernia": MR imaging findings. Radiology 2008;247(3):797–807.
18. Merskey H, Bogduk N. Classification of chronic pain: descriptions of chronic pain syndromes and definitions of pain terms. 2nd edition. Seattle (WA): IASP Press; 1994.
19. Choi H, McCartney M, Best TM. Treatment of osteitis pubis and osteomyelitis of the pubic symphysis in athletes: a systematic review. Br J Sports Med 2011;45(1):57–64.
20. O'Connell MJ, Powell T, McCaffrey NM, et al. Symphyseal cleft injection in the diagnosis and treatment of osteitis pubis in athletes. AJR Am J Roentgenol 2002;179(4):955–9.
21. Schwarzer AC, Aprill CN, Bogduk N. The sacroiliac joint in chronic low back pain. Spine (Phila Pa 1976) 1995;20(1):31–7.
22. Laslett M. Evidence-based diagnosis and treatment of the painful sacroiliac joint. J Man Manip Ther 2008;16(3):142–52.
23. Laslett M, Young SB, Aprill CN, et al. Diagnosing painful sacroiliac joints: a validity study of a McKenzie evaluation and sacroiliac provocation tests. Aust J Physiother 2003;49(2):89–97.
24. George SE, Clinton SC, Borello-France DF. Physical therapy management of female chronic pelvic pain: anatomic considerations. Clin Anat 2013;26(1):77–88.
25. Messing EM, Stamey TA. Interstitial cystitis: early diagnosis, pathology, and treatment. Urology 1978;12(4):381–92.

Pudendal Neuralgia

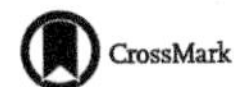

Waseem Khoder, MD, Douglass Hale, MD, FACOG, FACS*

KEYWORDS

- Pudendal neuralgia • Pudendal nerve entrapment • Nantes criteria
- Pudendal nerve block

KEY POINTS

- Pain is most often unilateral and increases with sitting.
- Diagnosis is made clinically. Nantes criteria can be helpful in making the diagnosis.
- Treatment options include physical therapy, medications, pudendal nerve blocks, and surgical decompression.

SYMPTOMS OF PUDENDAL NEURALGIA

Pudendal neuralgia is a painful neuropathic condition, involving the dermatome of the pudendal nerve.[1] Amarenco and colleagues[2,3] described pudendal neuralgia first in 1987. Patients with pudendal neuralgia usually present with burning pain in the distribution of the pudendal nerve. The pain is localized to the vulva, vagina, clitoris, perineum, and rectum in females and to the glans penis, scrotum, perineum, and rectum in males.[1] The pain can involve the entire area innervated by the pudendal nerve or affect a smaller region involving only a particular branch. In these cases, the pain is restricted to the terminal branches and may involve only the clitoris, the vulva/vaginal area alone, or the rectum alone.[4] Patients with pudendal neuralgia may have associated symptoms such as urinary frequency and urgency, symptoms of painful bladder syndrome, and dyspareunia.[5,6] The classic presentation of pudendal neuralgia is unilateral pain. However, bilateral pudendal neuralgia has been reported.[7]

Patients may have significant hyperalgesia (increased sensitivity and significant pain to mild painful stimulus), allodynia (pain in response to nonpainful stimulus), and paresthesias (sensation of tingling, pricking, or numbness).[7] Typically, symptoms are

The authors have nothing to disclose.
Division of Female Pelvic Medicine and Reconstructive Surgery, Department of Obstetrics and Gynecology, Indiana University School of Medicine, 1633 North Capitol Avenue, Suite 436, Indianapolis, IN 46202, USA
* Corresponding author.
E-mail address: dhale@iuhealth.org

Obstet Gynecol Clin N Am 41 (2014) 443–452
http://dx.doi.org/10.1016/j.ogc.2014.04.002 obgyn.theclinics.com
0889-8545/14/$ – see front matter

present when patients are sitting down and are much less severe or even absent when they lying down or standing.[4] Previous reports have shown that patients have significantly less pain when sitting on a toilet seat versus a chair. This phenomenon is believed to be associated with descent of the levator ani and less compression applied to the pudendal nerve. Patients usually awaken in the morning with minimal or no symptoms; however, the pain increases as the day progresses. Patients may report the sensation of having a foreign body in the vagina or feel as though they are sitting on an object. This pain may lead to some patients favoring a certain side while sitting, something that may be clinically observed by the clinician entering the examination room.[8]

ANATOMY

The pudendal nerve consists of sensory, motor, and autonomic nerve fibers. Sensory nerve cell bodies are located in the dorsal root ganglia of the sacrum, S2–S4. Anterior horn cells are located in the ventral horn of the sacral spinal cord (S2–S4) in a region called Onuf's (Onufrowicz) nucleus.[9] The nerve forms in the sacral plexus and comes to lie medially and caudally in relation to the trunk of the sciatic nerve. Passing laterally, it enters the gluteal region in the infrapiriform canal and then traverses the greater sciatic foramen.[1] Accompanied by its artery, usually situated cranial to the nerve, it is also surrounded by veins.

The pudendal bundle passes around the termination of the sacrospinous ligament just before its attachment to the ischial spine. At this level, the pudendal nerve is situated between the sacrospinous ligament ventrally and the sacrotuberous ligament dorsally. In rare cases, the nerve may travel between split layers of the sacrotuberous ligament. The nerve then passes ventrally, medially, and caudally and enters the perineal region via the lesser sciatic foramen. It lies lateral to the plane of the levator ani muscle traveling within a duplication of fascia on the medial surface of the obturator internus muscle, which forms the Alcock canal (**Fig. 1**).[10] The canal contains the pudendal nerve and vessels embedded in loose areolar tissue.[11] Most often, the 3 branches of the neurovascular bundle arise inside the canal: the inferior rectal nerve, the perineal nerve, and the dorsal nerve of the clitoris.[12]

The inferior rectal nerve supplies the integument around the anus and communicates with the perineal branch of the posterior femoral cutaneous nerve and its terminal branch, the labia majora nerve. The inferior rectal branch provides sensation to the distal aspect of the anal canal and to the perianal skin. This branch also provides motor innervation to the external anal sphincter.

The perineal nerve has a deep motor portion and 2 superficial sensory branches, the medial and lateral posterior labial nerves. This nerve provides sensation to the perineum and the ipsilateral labia majora. It also provides motor innervation to the transverse perinei muscle, the bulbospongiosus, the ischiocavernosus, and the sphincter urethrae and possibly contributes some branches to the levator ani muscles.[13] This branch emerges at the posterior part of the Alcock canal.[12]

The dorsal nerve of the clitoris is the terminal and most superficial branch of the pudendal nerve, found at the level of the symphysis pubis. The nerve is an afferent nerve that carries sensory information from the clitoris. Emerging from the dorsal aspect of the erectile organs, it travels in the infrapubic region and enters the Alcock canal where it joins the nerve trunk.[1]

Although the anatomy of the pudendal nerve is well outlined, great variation may exist, especially within the ischiorectal fossa, after its branches exit from Alcock

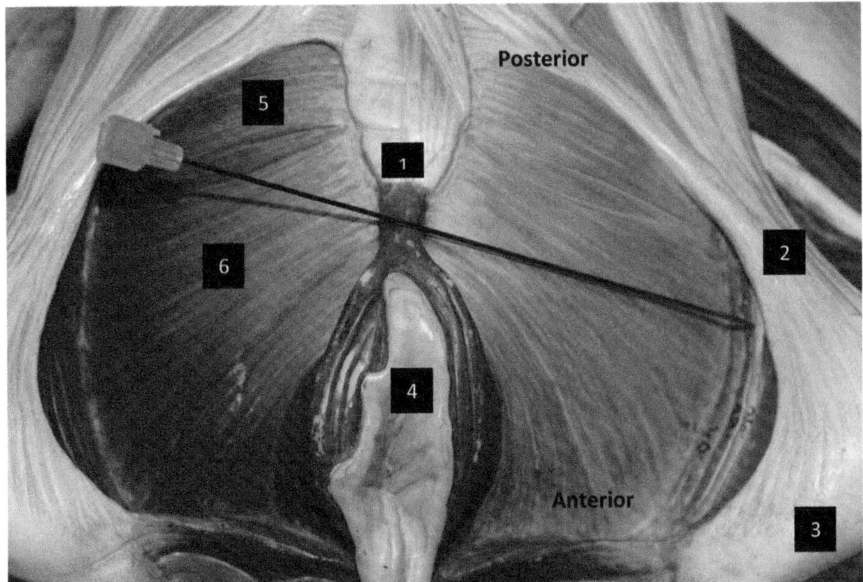

Fig. 1. The pudendal nerve (marked by a needle) when passing in the Alcock canal along the obturator internus muscle. 1, Coccyx; 2, sacrotuberous ligament; 3, ischial tuberosity; 4, anus; 5, piriformis muscle; 6, iliococcygeus muscle.

canal.[14] As the branches of the nerve run relatively superficially through the pelvis, they are vulnerable to injury.

CAUSES OF PUDENDAL NEURALGIA

Causes can be classified into mechanical, infectious, and immunologic.[15] The mechanical compromise may result from surgical procedures, trauma, or childbirth.[16] Mechanical compression has often been referred to as entrapment, similar to carpal tunnel syndrome.[17,18] This entrapment may be caused by pelvic floor muscle spasm, pressure from surrounding ligaments (sacrospinous, sacrotuberous), or scar tissue from trauma or surgeries involving the surrounding areas.

A common cause cited for entrapment is prior surgical procedure for prolapse or incontinence, where entrapment may be caused by mesh or suture.[19–21] Examples of procedures that have the potential to cause injury to the nerve are those that involve sacrospinous ligament fixation for the treatment of vaginal vault prolapse.[22,23] Because the nerve runs inferior to the sacrospinous ligament, there is the potential for entrapment of the nerve if the suture is misplaced.

Entrapment from inflammation and scarring can occur in patients with a prior history of pelvic trauma, falls injuring the back or buttocks, as well as traumatic insertion of foreign objects into the rectum or vagina. This scarring may occur around the ischial spine, between the sacrotuberous and sacrospinous ligaments, along the falciform process of the sacrotuberous ligament, or by compression of the nerve as it courses through Alcock canal.

Other causes may include herpes simplex infection, compression or inflammation from tumors, endometriosis, cycling, squatting exercises, and chemoradiation.[24–27]

NERVE INJURY TYPES

There are 3 common mechanisms of nerve injury:

1. Compression injuries are most common and can occur as acute or chronic lesions. The severity of damage is related to the magnitude as well as the duration of the trauma. Blood supply to the nerve is compromised, which may result in demyelination injury, and the resulting functional disorder may range from slight paresthesias and/or motor weakness to complete sensory loss and/or muscle paralysis.[28]
2. Stretch injuries can also occur and are commonly related to childbirth. As little as 10% stretch in relation to the length of the nerve can lead to damage.[29]
3. Transection injuries occur far less commonly, but are also most difficult to treat.[28]

Regeneration rates, including remyelination, have been reported to be around 1 mm/d in clinical situations, with further diminishing rates over time. These rates vary depending on the extent of injury, as well as the type, with higher rates of regeneration in compression injuries and lower rates in transection injuries.[30]

Classification of nerve injuries[31]:

Neurapraxia: trauma causes destruction of the myelin sheath, without affecting the axons or causing rupture of the surrounding connective tissue. This local conduction blockage resolves normally in less than 12 weeks as the nerve remyelinates.

Axonotmesis: trauma causes destruction of the myelin sheath and downstream Wallerian degeneration. The encapsulating connective tissue (endoneurium) is preserved, thus serving as a guide for proximal-distal axonal regrowth. Recovery is slow (1 mm/d) and usually complete.

Neurotmesis: there is a full transection of the nerve, with disrupted continuity in all the layers and downstream Wallerian degeneration. Surgical intervention to reestablish continuity is required, or nerve regrowth may result in a proximal neuroma.

DIAGNOSIS

History and physical examination are the most important components leading to diagnosis. Causes that can present with a similar constellation of symptoms must be excluded. These causes include painful bladder syndrome, vulvodynia, levator myalgia, piriformis syndrome, coccydynia, cauda equina syndrome, and neuralgias of other nerves such as the obturator, genitofemoral, or ilioinguinal nerves.

Detailed history should elicit the pain characteristics including onset, type, duration, aggravating and alleviating factors, and frequency. Examination should include inspection for any lesions in the perineum, vulva, and vagina; palpation and Q-tip examination to rule out vulvodynia; and bimanual examination focusing on pelvic floor muscles. In addition to the levator muscles, the piriformis and the obturator internus and externus should be thoroughly evaluated. Palpation on the ischial spine or pudendal nerve that produces paresthesias or pain is referred to Tinel's sign. Some patients start favoring one side of their pelvis while sitting, which can be discretely observed during history and physical examination.

Nantes Criteria for Diagnosis of Pudendal Neuralgia

In 2008, Dr Labat[4] published the Nantes criteria for the diagnosis of pudendal neuralgia.

This article gave some structure to making this diagnosis. According to these criteria, a patient must exhibit all 5 characteristics, without any symptoms of the exclusion criteria.[4]

Inclusion criteria

Nantes criteria for the diagnosis of pudendal neuralgia
Pain in the area innervated by the pudendal nerve extending from anus to clitoris
Pain is more severe when sitting
Pain does not awaken patients from sleep
Pain with no objective sensory impairment
Pain relieved by diagnostic pudendal block
Data from Labat JJ, Riant T, Robert R, et al. Diagnostic criteria for pudendal neuralgia by pudendal nerve entrapment (Nantes criteria). Neurourol Urodyn 2008;27(4):306–10.

Exclusion criteria

Pain located exclusively in the coccygeal, gluteal, pubic, or hypogastric area (without pain in the area of distribution of pudendal nerve)
Pruritus
Exclusively paroxysmal pain
Abnormalities on any imaging test (magnetic resonance imaging [MRI], computed tomography [CT], and others) that might explain the pain

Complementary diagnostic criteria

Pain characteristics: burning, shooting, stabbing, numbing
Allodynia or hyperesthesia
Sensation of foreign body in the rectum or vagina (sympathalgia)
Pain is progressively worse throughout the day
Pain is predominantly unilateral
Pain is triggered by defecation
Significant tenderness around the ischial spine on vaginal or rectal examination
Abnormal neurophysiology testing (pudendal nerve motor latency testing) in nulliparous women

Additional Testing

There are no imaging studies that diagnose pudendal neuralgia; however, MRI and CT may assist in excluding other causes of the pain.

Neurophysiology tests such as pudendal nerve terminal motor latency (PNTML) test and electromyography (EMG) may serve as complementary diagnostic measures.[32] However, they are not specific for patients with pudendal neuralgia. These tests can give abnormal results in multiple types of nerve injuries. This fact limits the utility of these tests when performed in multiparous women because of the high incidence of asymptomatic stretch and compression nerve injuries in this group of women.

In addition, PNTML test is a good test of demyelization and crushing but not of nerve fiber loss. The PNTML test examines only the motor function of the nerve and cannot provide any direct evidence of sensory nerve damage.[33] Therefore, an abnormal result of PNTML test indicates that the pudendal nerve is affected, but it is not specific for pudendal neuralgia. Conversely, a normal reading does not rule out pudendal neuralgia because only the motor nerves are being evaluated. During PNTML testing, the nerve is stimulated electrically and special electrodes measure the speed of the stimulus transmission. This speed includes the time for transmission along the axon from a designated spot on the nerve, transmission across the neuromuscular junction, and lastly, muscle contraction. If the latency in longer than 2.2 ms, nerve damage may be present. It should be noted that the PNTML measures only the largest, fastest conducting nerves. This measurement may remain normal despite extensive impairment of smaller nerves.[34]

EMG and single-fiber EMG with fiber density measurements are better able to document neuropathy compared with latency tests. However, this testing only evaluates the motor function of the nerve and can be quite uncomfortable and painful. To get useful results, multiple needle placements are required for recording data from the muscle. It is recommended that at least 20 sites be assessed and the results be averaged. The use of local anesthetic would adversely affect results.[35]

TREATMENT

Conservative Management

Physical therapy has been considered the first-line treatment by many investigators. Multiple stretches and exercises have been described to help reduce pain levels. Patients are preferably treated by therapists who specialize in pelvic floor therapy. Most of these patients have muscle spasm as a primary or secondary reaction. As such, therapists should address muscle imbalances, spasm, and other dysfunctions.[8] Therapists focus on palpation and manual techniques, posture, range of motion, and strength of the pelvis, back, and hips. Therapists have a variety of techniques to manually release the muscle spasm and help lengthen the muscles.[36] Therapy is most often applied through the vagina but can also be applied through the rectum.

Electrical stimulation and biofeedback have been used to assist therapists with treatment. Patients are given a home exercise regimen that includes relaxation and lifestyle modifications to continue the benefits gained during office sessions. In cases of muscle spasm refractory to physical therapy, botulinum toxin has been used.[37]

Medications can also be used for first-line treatment, including muscle relaxants and neuromodulators. Some of the medications commonly used are gabapentin, pregabalin (75 mg orally twice daily), cyclobenzaprine, and tricyclic antidepressants. Local medications, such as intravaginal diazepam (5-mg tablets up to 3 times daily or compounded suppositories), have also been applied; however, studies conflict on outcomes. Some studies mention using rectal belladonna and opium suppositories as possible adjuncts.[38]

Pudendal Nerve Block

Multiple approaches have been used for pudendal nerve block including transperineal, transgluteal, transrectal, and most often in women, a transvaginal approach. The ischial spine is used as a landmark to identify the injection site. CT-guided approaches have been reported in many studies. Investigators reported that using CT improves the accuracy of locating the pudendal nerve.[39] Another study reported fluoroscopy to aid in injection because the needle was placed on the tip of the ischial spine.[40] Magnetic resonance (MR) neurography has been used for the evaluation of some nerve compression syndromes including carpel tunnel syndrome and also applied to facilitate ulnar nerve release surgeries. It has been shown that MR neurography is as effective as needle EMG for identifying patients who are helped by surgical treatment. Filler[41] used MR neurography and open MR image-guided injections in a nonrandomized study in patients to distinguish different entrapment locations of the pudendal nerve.

Multiple injection protocols have been described using local anesthetics, steroids, or a combination of the two. One series offered a series of 3 CT-guided injections, each 6 weeks apart, using a combination of bupivacaine 0.5%, 5 mL, and triamcinolone 40 mg/mL, 2 mL.[38]

Another injection protocol described a set of 3 injections, each 1 week apart. The first injection is bupivacaine (3 mL of 0.25% solution) only with the next 2 injections being a mixture of methylprednisolone (1 mL 40 mg/mL solution) and bupivacaine (3 mL 0.25% solution), if the first one has provided relief to the patient. Immediate pain relief within minutes of therapy has been reported, and effects may last up to 6 weeks. Patients may benefit from repeated nerve blocks, and therapy needs to be individualized.[42]

Surgical Pudendal Nerve Decompression

Decompression is offered to patients when entrapment is suspected and pudendal nerve blocks have provided minimal or no relief. Approaches to decompression of an entrapped pudendal nerve include transgluteal, which is performed in the prone position, and those that may be approached from the lithotomy position. The latter includes the transperineal (also described as para-anal) and transvaginal approaches.

The transperineal approach involves opening Alcock canal through the ischiorectal fossa and releasing the nerve from its entrapment. Shafik[6] reported pain relief in 9 of 11 patients with pudendal neuralgia and vuvlvodynia. Beco and colleagues[43] used bilateral decompression through this approach for perineal pain and reported a 57% success rate.

The transgluteal approach uses a gluteal incision with the fibers of the gluteus muscle being separated longitudinally to reach the sacrotuberous ligament. The pudendal nerve is then identified after freeing and dividing the sacrotuberous ligament. The pudendal nerve is then decompressed along its entire length, from the piriformis muscle to Alcock canal. The fascia of the obturator internus muscle is incised, and the nerve is freed. The most common locations for pudendal nerve entrapment, as reported in the literature, are between the sacrospinous and sacrotuberous ligaments or the falciform process of sacrotuberous ligament.[44]

Hibner and colleagues[38] described their technique for pudendal nerve decompression in patients whom pudendal neuralgia began after sacrospinous ligament suspension or mesh-augmented surgery for prolapse. In these instances, suture or mesh material is often found directly entrapping the nerve. A segment of Neuragen (Origin Biomed Inc, Halifax, Canada) was used as a nerve-protecting tubing to prevent rescarring of the nerve. The nerve was also saturated with a platelet-rich plasma matrix, which has been shown to promote nerve healing in other nerve surgeries.[45] The sacrotuberous ligament was repaired with a graft of cadaveric gracilis tendon after placing a pain pump catheter along the course of the nerve. The catheter is removed at 20 days, and physical therapy started.[38]

Robert and colleagues[46] published the results of a prospective, randomized controlled trial that compared transgluteal decompression with nonsurgical treatment and repetitive pudendal blocks. A total of 32 patients were included in this study (16 in each group). After 1 year of treatment, 71.4% of the surgery group compared with 13.3% of the nonsurgery group showed improvement.

According to the literature, after surgical decompression, approximately 40% of patients are pain free, 30% have some improvement in pain, and 30% patients neither show improvement nor worsening.[46]

SUMMARY

Pudendal neuralgia is a painful condition affecting the nerve distribution of the pudendal nerve. The Nantes criteria give some structure in making the diagnosis for this frustrating condition. More research is needed to clarify the best diagnostic and treatment methods for this condition. Until then, a step-ladder approach to therapy, as described, is suggested when treating these patients.

REFERENCES

1. Robert R, Prat-Pradal D, Labat JJ, et al. Anatomic basis of chronic perineal pain: role of the pudendal nerve. Surg Radiol Anat 1998;20(2):93–8.
2. Amarenco G, Lanoe Y, Perrigot M, et al. A new canal syndrome: compression of the pudendal nerve in Alcock's canal or perinal paralysis of cyclists. Presse Med 1987;16(8):399 [in French].
3. Amarenco G, Savatovsky I, Budet C, et al. Perineal neuralgia and Alcock's canal syndrome. Ann Urol (Paris) 1989;23(6):488–92 [in French].
4. Labat JJ, Riant T, Robert R, et al. Diagnostic criteria for pudendal neuralgia by pudendal nerve entrapment (Nantes criteria). Neurourol Urodyn 2008;27(4): 306–10.
5. Waldinger MD, Venema PL, van Gils AP, et al. New insights into restless genital syndrome: static mechanical hyperesthesia and neuropathy of the nervus dorsalis clitoridis. J Sex Med 2009;6(10):2778–87.
6. Shafik A. Pudendal canal syndrome as a cause of vulvodynia and its treatment by pudendal nerve decompression. Eur J Obstet Gynecol Reprod Biol 1998;80(2): 215–20.
7. Ramsden CE, McDaniel MC, Harmon RL, et al. Pudendal nerve entrapment as source of intractable perineal pain. Am J Phys Med Rehabil 2003;82(6):479–84.
8. Benson JT, Griffis K. Pudendal neuralgia, a severe pain syndrome. Am J Obstet Gynecol 2005;192(5):1663–8.
9. Thor KB, Donatucci C. Central nervous system control of the lower urinary tract: new pharmacological approaches to stress urinary incontinence in women. J Urol 2004;172(1):27–33.
10. Juenemann KP, Lue TF, Schmidt RA, et al. Clinical significance of sacral and pudendal nerve anatomy. J Urol 1988;139(1):74–80.
11. Shafik A, el-Sherif M, Youssef A, et al. Surgical anatomy of the pudendal nerve and its clinical implications. Clin Anat 1995;8(2):110–5.
12. Shafik A, Doss S. Surgical anatomy of the somatic terminal innervation to the anal and urethral sphincters: role in anal and urethral surgery. J Urol 1999;161(1): 85–9.
13. Stein TA, DeLancey JO. Structure of the perineal membrane in females: gross and microscopic anatomy. Obstet Gynecol 2008;111(3):686–93.
14. Schraffordt SE, Tjandra JJ, Eizenberg N, et al. Anatomy of the pudendal nerve and its terminal branches: a cadaver study. ANZ J Surg 2004;74(1–2):23–6.
15. Marchand F, Perretti M, McMahon SB. Role of the immune system in chronic pain. Nat Rev Neurosci 2005;6(7):521–32.
16. Snooks SJ, Swash M, Mathers SE, et al. Effect of vaginal delivery on the pelvic floor: a 5-year follow-up. Br J Surg 1990;77(12):1358–60.

17. Pisani R, Stubinski R, Datti R. Entrapment neuropathy of the internal pudendal nerve. Report of two cases. Scand J Urol Nephrol 1997;31(4):407–10.
18. Antolak SJ Jr, Hough DM, Pawlina W, et al. Anatomical basis of chronic pelvic pain syndrome: the ischial spine and pudendal nerve entrapment. Med Hypotheses 2002;59(3):349–53.
19. Delmas V. Anatomical risks of transobturator suburethral tape in the treatment of female stress urinary incontinence. Eur Urol 2005;48(5):793–8.
20. Jelovsek JE, Sokol AI, Barber MD, et al. Anatomic relationships of infracoccygeal sacropexy (posterior intravaginal slingplasty) trocar insertion. Am J Obstet Gynecol 2005;193(6):2099–104.
21. Maher CF, Murray CJ, Carey MP, et al. Iliococcygeus or sacrospinous fixation for vaginal vault prolapse. Obstet Gynecol 2001;98(1):40–4.
22. Alevizon SJ, Finan MA. Sacrospinous colpopexy: management of postoperative pudendal nerve entrapment. Obstet Gynecol 1996;88(4 Pt 2):713–5.
23. Paraiso MF, Ballard LA, Walters MD, et al. Pelvic support defects and visceral and sexual function in women treated with sacrospinous ligament suspension and pelvic reconstruction. Am J Obstet Gynecol 1996;175(6):1423–30 [discussion: 1430–1].
24. Lim JF, Tjandra JJ, Hiscock R, et al. Preoperative chemoradiation for rectal cancer causes prolonged pudendal nerve terminal motor latency. Dis Colon Rectum 2006;49(1):12–9.
25. Howard EJ. Postherpetic pudendal neuralgia. JAMA 1985;253(15):2196.
26. Tognetti F, Poppi M, Gaist G, et al. Pudendal neuralgia due to solitary neurofibroma. Case report. J Neurosurg 1982;56(5):732–3.
27. Nehme-Schuster H, Youssef C, Roy C, et al. Alcock's canal syndrome revealing endometriosis. Lancet 2005;366(9492):1238.
28. Burnett MG, Zager EL. Pathophysiology of peripheral nerve injury: a brief review. Neurosurg Focus 2004;16(5):E1.
29. Henry MM, Swash M. Aetiology of pelvic floor disorders, in coloproctology and pelvic floor. Oxford (United Kingdom): Butterworth-Heinemann; 1992. p. 252–6.
30. Dagum AB. Peripheral nerve regeneration, repair, and grafting. J Hand Ther 1998;11(2):111–7.
31. HJ S. Brain, in three types of nerve injury. 1943. p. 237–88.
32. Olsen AL, Ross M, Stansfield RB, et al. Pelvic floor nerve conduction studies: establishing clinically relevant normative data. Am J Obstet Gynecol 2003;189(4): 1114–9.
33. Osterberg A, Graf W, Edebol Eeg-Olofsson K, et al. Results of neurophysiologic evaluation in fecal incontinence. Dis Colon Rectum 2000;43(9):1256–61.
34. Hill J, Hosker G, Kiff ES. Pudendal nerve terminal motor latency measurements: what they do and do not tell us. Br J Surg 2002;89(10):1268–9.
35. Gregory WT, Lou JS, Stuyvesant A, et al. Quantitative electromyography of the anal sphincter after uncomplicated vaginal delivery. Obstet Gynecol 2004; 104(2):327–35.
36. Amarenco G, Kerdraon J, Bouju P, et al. Treatments of perineal neuralgia caused by involvement of the pudendal nerve. Rev Neurol (Paris) 1997;153(5):331–4 [in French].
37. Abbott JA, Jarvis SK, Lyons SD, et al. Botulinum toxin type A for chronic pain and pelvic floor spasm in women: a randomized controlled trial. Obstet Gynecol 2006; 108(4):915–23.
38. Hibner M, Desai N, Robertson LJ, et al. Pudendal neuralgia. J Minim Invasive Gynecol 2010;17(2):148–53.

39. McDonald JS, Spigos DG. Computed tomography-guided pudendal block for treatment of pelvic pain due to pudendal neuropathy. Obstet Gynecol 2000; 95(2):306–9.
40. Choi SS, Lee PB, Kim YC, et al. C-arm-guided pudendal nerve block: a new technique. Int J Clin Pract 2006;60(5):553–6.
41. Filler AG. Diagnosis and treatment of pudendal nerve entrapment syndrome subtypes: imaging, injections, and minimal access surgery. Neurosurg Focus 2009;26(2):E9.
42. Stav K, Dwyer PL, Roberts L. Pudendal neuralgia. Fact or fiction? Obstet Gynecol Surv 2009;64(3):190–9.
43. Beco J, Climov D, Bex M. Pudendal nerve decompression in perineology: a case series. BMC Surg 2004;4:15.
44. Shafik A. Pudendal canal syndrome: a cause of chronic pelvic pain. Urology 2002;60(1):199.
45. Elgazzar RF, Mutabagani MA, Abdelaal SE, et al. Platelet rich plasma may enhance peripheral nerve regeneration after cyanoacrylate reanastomosis: a controlled blind study on rats. Int J Oral Maxillofac Surg 2008;37(8):748–55.
46. Robert R, Labat JJ, Bensignor M, et al. Decompression and transposition of the pudendal nerve in pudendal neuralgia: a randomized controlled trial and long-term evaluation. Eur Urol 2005;47(3):403–8.

Vulvodynia

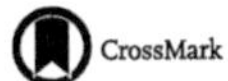

Mitul Shah, MD, Susan Hoffstetter, PhD, WHNP-BC*

KEYWORDS

• Vulvodynia • Vulvar pain • Vaginismus

KEY POINTS

- Vulvodynia is a chronic pain disorder.
- Cause is considered to be multifactorial.
- Evaluation and diagnosis is key to appropriate management.
- Therapies include self-management and nonpharmacologic, pharmacologic, and surgical treatment.
- Emotional and psychological support is invaluable.
- Vaginismus occurs commonly with vulvodynia.

DIAGNOSIS

Introduction

Vulvodynia has been described since the 1880s as an "excessive sensibility of the nerves supplying the mucous membranes of the vulva"[1] or "supersensitivities of the vulva."[2] It was described as "burning vulvar syndrome" by the International Society for the Study of Vulvovaginal Disease (ISSVD) in 1975. A variety of terms have been used to label vulvar pain, including *essential vulvodynia*, *dysesthetic vulvodynia*, *vulvar vestibulitis syndrome*, *vulvar dysesthesia*, *provoked vulvar dysesthesias*, or *spontaneous vulvar dysesthesia*. In 2003, the ISSVD settled on the current classification of generalized or localized, and then each type subdivided into provoked, unprovoked, or mixed.[3]

Definition

Chronic vulvar pain lasting 3 months or longer is termed *vulvodynia*. The ISSVD defines vulvodynia as chronic vulvar discomfort or pain, characterized by burning, stinging, irritation, or rawness of the female genitalia in which there is no infection, skin disease, or neoplasia of the vulva or vagina, or specific clinically identifiable neurologic disorder as the cause of these symptoms.[4]

The authors have nothing to disclose.
Department of Obstetrics Gynecology & Women's Health, Saint Louis University School of Medicine, 6420 Clayton Road, St Louis, MO 63117, USA
* Corresponding author.
E-mail address: hoffstes@slu.edu

Obstet Gynecol Clin N Am 41 (2014) 453–464
http://dx.doi.org/10.1016/j.ogc.2014.05.005 **obgyn.theclinics.com**
0889-8545/14/$ – see front matter

The classification of vulvodynia is based on the site of the pain, whether it is localized or generalized, and whether the pain is provoked, unprovoked, or mixed.[5] *Provoked* refers to any touch or stimulation that elicits pain, sexual or nonsexual. *Unprovoked* refers to pain that occurs in the absence of touch or stimulation, and *mixed* refers to pain that varies with or without touch or stimulation. Localized and generalized vulvodynia can be provoked, unprovoked, or mixed.

Localized vulvodynia or vestibulodynia is pain that is caused by touching a localized area of the vulva, commonly occurring in the region of the vestibular glands. It can also occur at the clitoris, clitorodynia or on one side of the vulva, hemivulvodynia. The pain has been described as a feeling of burning, stinging, tearing, throbbing, razor blades, or cut glass. Women with localized vulvodynia have dyspareunia or avoid sex, because of the pain at the introitus. The pain can last for hours to days after sexual touch, intercourse, or attempts at intercourse. Inserting or wearing tampons can be painful. Women may not be able to engage in routine exercise or activities, such as riding a bicycle or wearing tight clothing or jeans. Patients can be pain-free if the painful areas are not touched. Localized vulvodynia is further subdivided into primary, vestibular pain during the first attempt at vaginal penetration versus secondary, and vestibular pain after a period of normal function. A recent study showed that primary and secondary vulvodynia had different histologic features, indicating they may be different entities.[6]

Generalized vulvodynia is pain and burning on or around the vulva, including the mons pubis, labia majora, labia minora, vestibule, and perineum. Women with generalized vulvodynia describe burning, stinging, rawness, and aching in the vulva. The pain may be constant or intermittent. It may range from mild discomfort to severe pain that can prevent daily activities. Symptoms may be diffuse or in different areas at different times. Some days the pain may be less than others, but the area hurts most of the time, even when nothing is touching it. Sitting may be uncomfortable. Some women report increased vaginal discharge with the pain. Urination may contribute to the pain and burning. Sexual touch or intercourse is occasionally possible for some women.

Symptoms and Prevalence

Vulvodynia affects women of all age groups, from adolescence through menopause.[7] Common vulvar symptoms reported include burning, stinging, rawness, itching, aching, soreness, or throbbing of the vulvar tissues. Pain may be constant, intermittent, localized, or diffuse. Symptoms may occur during intercourse and exercise, or even while sitting or resting. A study by Sadownik[8] found that women presented with symptoms including dyspareunia (71%), history of recurrent yeast infection (64%), vulvar burning (57%), vulvar itching (46%), and problems with sexual response (33%).[9] Repeated urogenital infections, such as bacterial vaginosis, candidiasis, condyloma, trichomoniasis, and urinary tract infections, have been shown to be a risk factor for the development of vulvodynia. Multiple infections compound the risk of vulvodynia, with an odds ratio greater than 8 for 3 or more infections reported in the 12 months before the onset of vulvodynia.[10]

Vulvodynia causes significant physical and psychological distress and affects quality of life. Vulvodynia is diagnosed through exclusion. The prevalence of vulvodynia is approximately 8.3% to 16.0% of women in the United States.[9,11] A National Institutes of Health study estimates that 13 million women may experience symptoms at some point in their lifetime[12] and that 6% of women have symptoms before the age of 25 years.[7] These prevalence rates are believed to be greatly underreported because of the absence of visible abnormalities of the vulva.

Etiology

The cause of vulvodynia is unknown. Theories suggest a multifactorial origin, including embryonic derivation,[12,13] chronic inflammation,[14] genetic immune factors,[15,16] nerve pathways,[17–20] abnormal response to environmental factors (eg, infection, irritants, trauma), hormonal changes,[21] human papilloma virus, and oxalates.[22,23] The pathophysiology suggests that vulvodynia is a chronic disorder of the nerves that supply the vulva. The painful tissue has been shown to have nerve fiber proliferation or neural hyperplasia.[17–19] Chronic inflammation, such as is caused by contact irritants, recurrent vulvovaginal infections, hormonal changes, and chronic skin conditions, acts as a trigger. Normal sensations are perceived as abnormal, which results in heightened sensitivity.

Comorbidities with Psychological Diagnosis and Chronic Pain Conditions

A relationship has been shown between comorbid pain conditions. In a study by Reed and colleagues,[24] approximately 1940 women were screened for interstitial cystitis, irritable bowel syndrome, fibromyalgia, and vulvodynia. Prevalence ranged from 7.5% to 11.8%. However, 27% screened positive for multiple conditions. The presence of vulvodynia was significantly associated with other pain syndromes ($P<.001$), with an odds ratio of 2.3 to 3.3. Other associated conditions include recurrent yeast infections and chronic fatigue syndrome.[25,26]

The chronic nature of vulvodynia can negatively affect a woman's self-image and lead to psychological disorders, such as depression and anxiety. Vulvodynia is not considered a psychopathological condition.[7,27] However, in a study by Tribo and colleagues,[28] more than 50% of women report depression and/or anxiety as a presenting symptom. Further studies have shown that the odds of having vulvodynia are 4 times more likely in women with antecedent mood or anxiety disorders.[29] Vulvodynia has also been associated with new or recurrent mood and anxiety disorders, with an odds ratio of 1.7.[29]

Women presenting with vulvodynia may also experience significant sexual, psychological, and relationship problems. Many may benefit from psychological support, sex therapy, and/or counseling. The cycle of pain caused by vulvodynia may ultimately lead to avoidance of all sexual activities; fear of pain and anticipation of pain during sexual intercourse may lead to partial avoidance of sexual intimacy and activity, sexual arousal disorder, loss of libido, problems with orgasm/anorgasmic disorders, phobic avoidance of sexual activities, and subsequent relationship difficulties.

Evaluation and Physical Examination

Evaluation of the patient with vulvodynia should include a comprehensive medical history, noting any association of life changes, stressors, new medical conditions, childbirth and lactation, menopausal status, surgeries, and previous failed therapies with the onset of symptoms or symptom flares. Identification of possible contact irritants through patient recall includes all products that come in contact with the vulvar skin. This identification is critical to optimize the condition of the vulvar tissues. Common irritants include scented detergents, soaps, and over-the-counter feminine hygiene products.

The vulva should be inspected for any abnormalities, including dermatoses and premalignant or malignant conditions. If any abnormal or suspicious conditions are identified, a biopsy or vulvar colposcopy is indicated and appropriate referral or treatment performed. In the absence of abnormal dermatologic findings other than erythema, a vulvar colposcopy has limited value.[30]

Cotton swab testing should be used to identify painful areas on the vulva or areas that are symptomatic (**Fig. 1**). The cotton swap should be touched lightly in a consistent pattern starting with the outer thighs, mons, labia majora, inner labia folds, labia minora, posterior fourchette, and vestibule, and in the region of the periurethral and Bartholin glands. For the vestibule, left and right sides should be examined separately rather than trying to spread the labia and examine both sides at once. Patients should be instructed to either classify areas as painless, or having mild, moderate, or severe pain, or apply a number value based on a Likert 10-point pain scale (ranging from 0 = none to 10 = most severe level of pain). Localized vulvodynia can be diagnosed if the patient experiences discrete areas of pain, and generalized vulvodynia can be diagnosed if the patient experiences pain in a broad area. If no pain, tenderness, or burning is elicited with cotton swab testing, vulvodynia would not be considered in the differential diagnosis.[5]

Vaginal examination should be performed, including a wet mount analysis and yeast culture. Infectious or inflammatory diseases should be ruled out, such as candidiasis, recurrent vaginitis, herpes simplex virus, and a desquamative inflammatory vaginitis. Normal findings such as atrophy should be considered in lactating or perimenopausal to postmenopausal populations. A speculum examination is not always required, because a cotton swab inserted vaginally is adequate to collect a specimen for wet mount analysis. A yeast culture is the gold standard for identifying yeast and offers species identification with drug sensitivities to guide treatment.[31] The yeast culture can be obtained from areas on the labia and vestibule, and from the vaginal canal. Any abnormal conditions identified should be treated.

Vaginismus, or involuntary spasm of the pelvic floor muscles, is a common finding with vulvodynia. Evaluation and management are necessary to improve patient outcomes.[32] To test for vaginismus, pressure with a gloved finger should be applied to the levator ani and obturator internus muscles. If pressure elicits tenderness or pain, and/or muscles are in a state of contracture, vaginismus can be diagnosed.

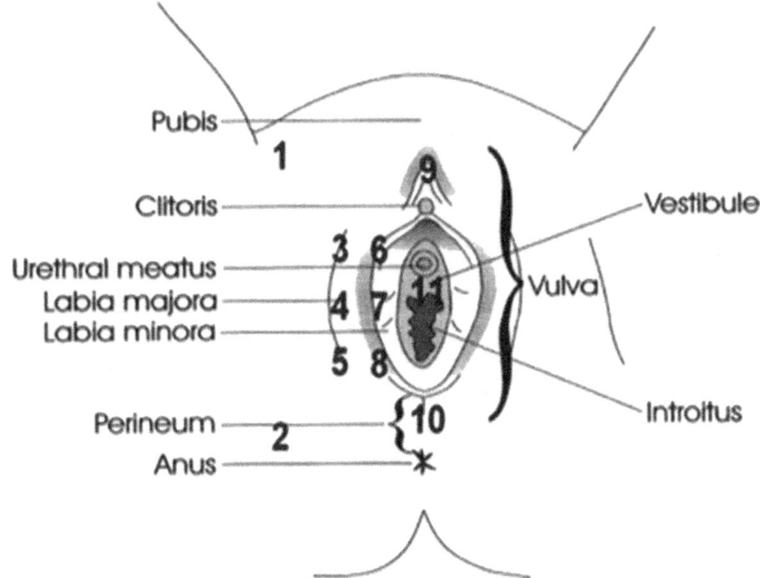

Fig. 1. Cotton swab testing. Check clockwise: 1–2, inner thigh; 3–5, labia majora; 6–8, interlabial sulcus; 9, clitoris and hood; 10, perineum; 11, vestibule.

TREATMENT

Management Goals

Vulvodynia is a chronic pain condition that presents management challenges for clinicians and patients. Symptom resolution is not often a realistic outcome. The primary goals of treatment are symptom reduction, improvement in quality of life and sexual function, and return to activities of daily living. Patient understanding and acceptance of treatment goals is critical. Treatments can be slow and frustrating because just as there is no single cause for vulvodynia, there is no single treatment that is effective for symptom relief for all women.

In 2006, the American College of Obstetricians and Gynecologists published Committee Opinion #345 on vulvodynia, which stated a few important points for practitioners to remember when treating patients with vulvodynia:

Most available evidence for the treatment of vulvodynia is based on clinical experience, descriptive studies, or reports of expert committees.
Few randomized controlled trials have been conducted of vulvodynia treatments.
Vulvodynia is a complex disorder that is difficult to treat, and rapid resolution is unusual, even with proper treatment.
A decrease in pain may take weeks to months and may not be complete.
No single treatment is successful in all women.[33]

Initial treatment steps must include self-management strategies to maximize tissue quality and eliminate possible contributing factors for vulvar pain. The addition of pharmacologic agents, as tolerated in increasing dosages and combinations, is needed to maximize the response. Nonpharmacologic approaches are equally important to offer holistic care to these women.

Self-Management Strategies

Education regarding the implementation of strict vulvar care/hygiene is essential to eliminate the possibility of contact irritants as a cause or trigger for vulvar symptoms. Adherence to vulvar hygiene has been shown to be an effective initial strategy to reduce vulvar complaints of burning, itching, pain, and dyspareunia.[34] Dyes, perfumes, or enzymes in any product that come in contact with the vulvar tissues should be considered a source of irritation, including laundry detergents, fabric softeners, body soaps, feminine hygiene products, noncotton underwear, and over-the-counter vaginal products.[33]

To reduce symptoms, bathing the vulva in a mild baking soda solution can be soothing; this is a simple treatment that patients can use to attenuate their symptoms that does not require the use of medications. Lukewarm water is recommended, because hot water can exacerbate vulvar symptoms. Caution should be exercised if using the bathtub for the sitz bath, because residue from cleaning products can serve as a contact irritant. Ice packs applied to the vulva for 2 to 3 minutes at a time can offer relief without harm.[5] To improve the quality of the vulvar skin, vegetable oil or olive oil serves as an emollient. These substances can be used liberally and often for comfort and to reduce symptoms. A&D ointment and zinc oxide serve to form a barrier to protect the skin and can be applied twice a day as necessary.

Pharmacologic Strategies

In selecting a vehicle for delivery of topical medications, ointments provide a better mode of delivery, minimizing the risk of causing a flare of symptoms. Creams contain

Table 1
Pharmacologic agents for vulvodynia

	Name	Dose	Side Effects	Comments
Topical medications	Lidocaine 5% ointment	Apply as needed in small amount Systemic absorption possible with frequent or excessive use	Erythema	Temporary relief before coitus; short-term use only
	Doxepin 5% cream in water-soluble base	Apply to skin once daily, with gradual increase, not to exceed 4 times daily		
	Gabapentin 2%–6% in water-soluble base			
	Amitriptyline 2% with baclofen 2% in water-soluble base	Apply 1–3 times daily	Irritation, erythema, rash	Topical formulation has fewer side effects than systemic
Oral neuropathic pain modulators				
Antidepressants	Amitriptyline	10 mg nightly & increase by 10 mg q3–4 wk Maximum dose 150 mg qd	Drowsiness, dizziness dry mouth, constipation, weight gain, urinary retention, tachycardia, blurred vision, confusion	Have patients avoid more than one drink of alcohol each day Advise contraception Consider lower doses in elderly (over age 65) patients
	Desipramine	Same dosing as amitriptyline	Drowsiness, dizziness, blurred vision, dry mouth, constipation, tachycardia, urinary retention, diaphoresis, weakness, nervousness, rash seizures, tinnitus, anxiety, confusion	
	Duloxetine	Start with 30 mg qd bid		No data to support its use
	Venlafaxine	Start with 37.5 mg Maximum 150 mg qd	Headache, nausea, somnolence, weight loss, anorexia, constipation, anxiety, vision changes, diarrhea, dizziness, dry mouth, insomnia, weakness, sweating, hypertension	Few data to support use

Anticonvulsants	Gabapentin	Start with 100–300 mg at nightly & advance as tolerated in divided dose bid to tid Common doses range from 300–1800 mg Maximum dose, 3600 mg Maximum dose, 1200 mg in a single dose	Dizziness, somnolence, ataxia, fatigue, nystagmus, tremor, diplopia, rhinitis, blurred vision, nausea, vomiting, nervousness, dysarthria, weight gain	
	Pregabalin	Start with 50–75 mg Common doses range from 75–150 mg Maximum dose, 600 mg bid	Dizziness, peripheral edema, weight gain, somnolence	Faster onset; however, may be less tolerated than gabapentin
Other agents	Topiramate	Use only after previously mentioned therapies unsuccessful Start at 25 mg qd bid Maximum dose, 200 mg bid	Dose-related Fatigue, paresthesia, tremor, asthenia, confusion, dizziness, diplopia, difficult concentration, memory problems, nervousness	Few data to support use Interferes with hormonal contraception
	Lamotrigine	Use after previously mentioned therapies unsuccessful		One clinical trial to support its use Interferes with hormonal contraception
	Hydroxyzine	25 mg to reduce pruritus		
	Cetirizine	10 mg to reduce pruritus		

more preservatives and stabilizers, which can act as contact irritants and cause burning on application.[5]

Topical Medications

Local anesthetics, such as lidocaine ointment, can provide temporary relief from the pain to enable intercourse, if applied topically to the vulva a few minutes before coitus. In 2003, Zolnoun and colleagues[35] advised overnight use of topical lidocaine to allow for healing, and reported that women experienced a significant decrease in pain with sexual activity. Benzocaine is not advised because it can produce contact irritation and may cause a flare-up of symptoms.[36] The use of topical antidepressants, such as doxepin 5% cream, gabapentin 2% to 6%, or amitriptyline 2% mixed with baclofen 2% in a water-washable base can be applied by fingertip to the affected areas.[36]

Pain Medications

Narcotic pain medications should be used with caution in patients with vulvodynia. Tramadol and hydrocodone/acetaminophen combinations have been used in the short term for vulvodynia flares.

Pain Modulators

The use of neuropathic pain modulators, including tricyclic antidepressants such as amitriptyline or desipramine can help decrease neuropathic chronic pain through a central action altering the transmission of pain impulses to the brain through the dorsal horn.[37] In a small National Institute of Child Health and Human Development–funded study, amitriptyline with or without topical triamcinolone was no more effective than self-management approaches in managing vulvar pain.[38] A randomized controlled trial showed that oral desipramine and topical lidocaine, alone or in combination, were not superior to placebo.[39] Other antidepressants, such as duloxetine and venlafaxine, have also been used, but few data support their use. A randomized controlled trial is currently evaluating the use of gabapentin, a drug that helps control epileptic seizures, for women with provoked vestibulodynia.[40]

The newest anticonvulsant used for chronic pain is pregabalin. A small retrospective chart review showed improvement in symptoms (Aranda J, Edwards L, unpublished data, 2007). A small open-label trial with lamotrigine has shown a decrease in pain at 8 weeks.[41] Topiramate has also been used, but few supportive data are available. Hydroxyzine and cetirizine have been used to reduce pruritis. For some women, combinations of neuropathic pain medications (eg, amitriptyline, gabapentin, and pregabalin) can also be used, because they have different mechanisms of action. Neuropathic pain medications should not be stopped suddenly; dosages should be weaned before discontinuation (**Table 1**).

Nonpharmacologic Strategies

Nonpharmacologic strategies can be used as an adjunct to any of the therapies mentioned earlier. Psychological treatment can provide techniques for relaxation or coping with pain or an opportunity to explore other conditions that may relate to the pain.[5] Couples therapy and sexual therapy are additional options that may benefit both the patient and partner. A randomized, controlled trial found that women who had cognitive behavioral therapy reported a 30% decrease in vulvar pain that occurs with intercourse.[42]

Limited research has been performed on hypnotherapy for vulvodynia.[43] A case report showed resolution of localized vulvodynia after 12 psychotherapy sessions, 8 of which included hypnosis. Some small pilot studies have shown that acupuncture treatment for localized vulvodynia was well tolerated, and that quality-of-life measurements were higher after completing treatment and at 3-month follow-up.[44–46]

An association between oxalates and vulvar pain has been theorized. High levels of oxalate in the urine can be reduced with diet and calcium citrate, although little evidence exists to support the use or effectiveness of this treatment for vulvar pain.[23]

Surgery

Surgical excision of the vulvar vestibule (ie, vestibulectomy) for women with localized vulvodynia is an option chosen cautiously after failure of other attempted therapies. Success rates vary from 60% to 85% at short-term follow-up.[47–49] The area of excision is outlined in **Fig. 2**. Neuropathic pain medications are usually continued postoperatively to maximize quality of life and promote return of sexual functioning.[36]

Vaginismus

Vaginismus may develop subsequent to any chronic pelvic pain condition and is common with vulvodynia. Assessment for and treatment of this condition is critical, because it may be the cause of continued pain and/or sexual dysfunction after successful treatment of vulvodynia.

Nonpharmacologic Strategies

Nonpharmacologic treatment for vaginismus includes physical therapy with pelvic floor exercises and biofeedback. Patient control of specific body responses enables relaxation of pelvic muscles, resulting in subsequent pain reduction. The authors' clinical experience has found increased success, with lower cotton swab pain scores at initiation of physical therapy. Physical therapists must be specifically trained in pelvic floor and biofeedback for optimum results. Success rates of 60% to 80% have been reported with pelvic floor–trained physical therapists.[50]

Vaginal dilators can be helpful to overcome tension in the pelvic floor muscles and are available in varying sizes. Patient's can use the dilator before attempting intercourse to accommodate penetration when symptoms allow a return to sexual activity. Hypnosis[43] has been used with some limited success.

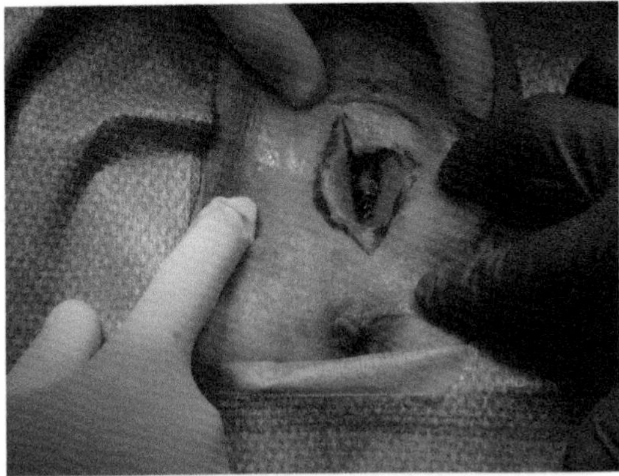

Fig. 2. Surgical excision of the vulvar vestibule, vestibulectomy.

Pharmacologic Strategies

Pharmacologic treatments include vaginal valium inserted at bedtime and topical baclofen. Research studies are ongoing with Botox injections.[51,52]

SUMMARY AND DISCUSSION

Vulvodynia causes significant physical and psychological distress and impacts quality of life in women and their families. Patients with vulvodynia often seek care from many providers, attempting to find resolution of their symptoms. A prospective study of 300 patients showed that 60% of women consulted 3 or more physicians in seeking a diagnosis, and 40% remained undiagnosed.[8] Spontaneous remission has occurred in some women, but most have had multiple attempts with medical management without 100% resolution of symptoms. Referral to vaginal and vulvar disease clinics should be encouraged to optimize management strategies and maximize quality of life for these patients and their partners. Concurrent emotional and psychological support can be invaluable.

REFERENCES

1. Thomas TG. Practical treatise on the diseases of women. Philadelphia: Henry C Leason; 1880. p. 145.
2. Skene AJ. Diseases of the external organs of generation. In: Treatise on the Diseases of Women. New York: D Appleton & Co; 1888. p. 77–99.
3. Moyal-Barracco M, Lynch PJ. 2003 ISSVD terminology and classification of vulvodynia: a historical perspective. J Reprod Med 2004;49(10):772–7.
4. Haefner HK. Report of the ISSVD terminology and classification of vulvodynia. J Low Genit Tract Dis 2007;11(1):4809 ISSVD.
5. Haefner HK, Collins ME, Davis GD, et al. The vulvodynia guideline. J Low Genit Tract Dis 2005;9:40–51.
6. LeClair C, Goetsch M, Korcheva V, et al. Differences in primary compared with secondary vestibulodynia by immunohistochemistry. Obstet Gynecol 2011; 117(6):1307–13.
7. Metts JF. Vulvodynia and vulvar vestibulitis: challenges in diagnosis and management. Am Fam Physician 1999;59:1547–56, 1561–2.
8. Sadownik LA. Clinical profile of vulvodynia patients. A prospective study of 300 patients. J Reprod Med 2000;45:679–84.
9. Harlow BL, Stewart EG. A population-based assessment of chronic unexplained vulvar pain: have we underestimated the prevalence of vulvodynia? J Am Med Womens Assoc 2003;58:82–8.
10. Nguyen RH, Swanson D, Harlow BL. Urogenital infections in relation to the occurrence of vulvodynia. J Reprod Med 2009;54(6):385–92.
11. Reed BD, Harlow SD, Sen A, et al. Prevalence and demographic characteristics of vulvodynia in a population based sample. Am J Obstet Gynecol 2012;206(2): 170.e1–9.
12. McCormack WM. Two urogenital sinus syndromes. Interstitial cystitis and focal vulvitis. J Reprod Med 1990;35(9):873–6.
13. Fitzpatrick CC, DeLancey JO, Elkins TE, et al. Vulvar vestibulitis and interstitial cystitis; a disorder of urogenital sinus-derived epithelium. Obstet Gynecol 1993;81(5):860–2.
14. Sloan S, Reynold L, Gall S, et al. Chronic inflammation in vestibular tissue is normal. Int J Gynecol Pathol 1999;18:360–6.

15. Goetsch MF. Vulvar vestibulitis: prevalence and historic features in a general gynecologic practice population. Am J Obstet Gynecol 1991;164(6 Pt 1):1609–14 [discussion: 1614–6].
16. Foster DC, Piekarz KH, Murant TI, et al. Enhanced synthesis of pro inflammatory cytokines by vulvar vestibular fibroblasts: implications for vulvar vestibulitis. Am J Obstet Gynecol 2007;196(4):346.e1–8.
17. Bohm-Starke N, Hilliges M, Falconer C, et al. Increased intraepithelial innervation in women with vulvar vestibulitis syndrome. Gynecol Obstet Invest 1998; 46(4):256–60.
18. Tympanidis P, Terenghi G, Dowd P. Increased innervation of the vulvar vestibule in patients with vulvodynia. Br J Dermatol 2003;148(5):1021–7.
19. Weström LV, Willén R. Vestibular nerve fiber proliferation in vulvar vestibulitis syndrome. Obstet Gynecol 1998;91(4):572–6.
20. Krantz KE. Innervation of the human vulva and vagina. Obstet Gynecol 1959;12: 382–96.
21. Eva LJ, MacLean AB, Reid WM, et al. Estrogen receptor expression. Am J Obstet Gynecol 2003;189:458–61.
22. Greenstein A, Militscher I, Chen J, et al. Hyperoxaluria in women with vulvar vestibulitis syndrome. J Reprod Med 2006;51(6):500–2.
23. Harlow BL, Abenhaim HA, Vitonis AF, et al. Influence of dietary oxalates on the risk of adult onset vulvodynia. J Reprod Med 2008;53(3):171–8.
24. Reed BD, Harlow SD, Sen A, et al. Relationship between vulvodynia and chronic comorbid pain conditions. Obstet Gynecol 2012;120(1):145–51.
25. Gardella B, Parru D, Nappi R, et al. Interstitial cystitis is associated with vulvodynia and sexual dysfunction a case control study. J Sex Med 2011;8(6):1726–34.
26. Carric D, Shere K, Peters K. The relationship of interstitial cystitis/painful bladder syndrome to vulvodynia. Urol Nurs 2009;29(4):233–8.
27. Bornstein J, Zarfati D, Abramovici H. Vulvar vestibulitis: physical or psychosexual problem? Obstet Gynecol 1999;93:876–80.
28. Tribo MJ, Andio O, Ros S, et al. Clinical characteristics and psychopathological profile of patients with vulvodynia: an observational and descriptive study. Dermatology 2008;216(1):24–30.
29. Khandker M, Brady SS, Vitonis AF, et al. The influence of depression and anxiety on risk of adult onset vulvodynia. J Womens Health (Larchmt) 2011;20(10): 1445–51.
30. Balgia BS, editor. Principles & practice of colposcopy. New Delhi (India): JP Medical Pub; 2011. p. 195–206.
31. Geiger AM, Foxman B, Sobel J. Chronic vulvovaginal candidiasis: characteristics of women with candida albicans, candida glabrata and no candida. Genitourin Med 1995;71(5):304–7.
32. Abramov L, Wolman I, David MP, et al. Vaginismus: an important factor in the evaluation and management of vulvar vestibulitis syndrome. Gynecol Obstet Invest 1994;38(3):194–7.
33. American College of Obstetricians and Gynecologists. Committee opinion number 345 October 2006. Vulvodynia. Washington, DC: American College of Obstetricians and Gynecologists; 2006.
34. Lifits-Podorozhansky YM, Podorozhansky Y, Hoffstetter S, et al. Role of vulvar care guidelines in the initial management of vulvar complaints. J Low Genit Tract Dis 2012;16(2):88–91.
35. Zolnoun DA, Hartmann KE, Steege JF. Overnight lidocaine ointment for treatment of vulvar vestibulitis. Obstet Gynecol 2003;102:84–7.

36. Edwards L. Vulvovaginal pain causes and management. Vulvovaginal disease update 2013. Durham, May 31, 2013.
37. Reed BD, Caron AM, Gorenflo DW, et al. Treatment of vulvodynia with tricyclic antidepressants: efficacy and associated factors. J Low Genit Tract Dis 2006; 10(4):245–51.
38. Brown CS, Wan J, Bachmann G, et al. Self-management, amitriptyline, and amitriptyline plus triamcinolone in the management of vulvodynia. J Womens Health (Larchmt) 2009;18:163–9.
39. Foster DC, Kotok MB, Huang LS, et al. Oral desipramine and topical lidocaine for vulvodynia: a randomized controlled trial. Obstet Gynecol 2010;116:583–93.
40. Brown C. A trial of gabapentin in vulvodynia: biological correlates of response. University of Tennessee. NIH Project. 8/2012-3/2015.
41. Meltzer-Brody SE, Zolnoun D, Steege JF, et al. Open label trial of lamotrigine focusing on efficacy in vulvodynia. J Reprod Med 2009;54:171–8.
42. Bergeron S, Binik YM, Khalifé S, et al. A randomized comparison of group cognitive-behavioral therapy, surface electromyographic biofeedback, and vestibulectomy in the treatment of dyspareunia resulting from vulvar vestibulitis. Pain 2001;91:297–306.
43. Kandyba K, Binik YM. Hypnotherapy as a treatment for vulvar vestibulitis syndrome: a case report. J Sex Marital Ther 2003;29:237–42.
44. Danielsson I, Sjorg I, Ostman C. Acupuncture for the treatment of vulvar vestibulitis: a pilot study. Acta Obstet Gynecol Scand 2001;80:437–41.
45. Aung SK. Sexual dysfunction: a modern medical acupuncture approach. Medical Acupuncture 2002;13(2):7–9.
46. Powell J, Wojinarowska F. Acupuncture for vulvodynia. J R Soc Med 1999;92: 579–81.
47. McCormack WM, Spence M. Evaluation of the surgical treatment for vulvar vestibulitis. Eur J Obstet Gynecol Reprod Biol 1999;86:135–8.
48. Haefner HK. Critique of new gynecologic surgical procedures: surgery for vulvar vestibulitis. Clin Obstet Gynecol 2000;43:689–700.
49. Goldstein A, Klingman D, Christopher K, et al. Surgical treatment of vulvar vestibulitis syndrome: outcome assessment derived from a postoperative questionnaire. J Sex Med 2006;3:923–31.
50. Haefner HK. Vulvovaginal disease update 2013. Vulvodynia. Durham, May 31, 2013.
51. Pelletier F, Parratte B, Penz S, et al. Efficacy of high doses of botulinum toxin A for treating of provoked vestibulodynia. Br J Dermatol 2011;164:617–22.
52. Petersen CD, Giraldi A, Lundvall L, et al. Botulinum toxin type A-a novel treatment for provoked vestibulodynia? Results from a randomized placebo controlled double blinded study. J Sex Med 2009;9:2523–37.

Gastrointestinal Causes of Abdominal Pain

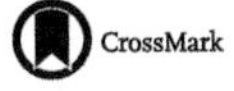

Elizabeth Marsicano, MD*, Giao Michael Vuong, MD, Charlene M. Prather, MD, MPH, AGAF, FACP*

KEYWORDS

• Abdominal pain • Epigastric pain • RUQ pain • LUQ pain • RLQ pain • LLQ pain • Nausea • Vomiting

KEY POINTS

- Gastrointestinal (GI) causes of abdominal pain are numerous.
- GI causes of abdominal pain can be divided into acute abdominal pain and chronic abdominal pain.
- Subcategorization by location of pain as it pertains to the abdomen can aid in understanding root causes.

INTRODUCTION

A complaint of abdominal pain remains among the most common symptoms that bring a patient to medical attention. The differential diagnosis varies greatly between acute abdominal pain and chronic abdominal pain. Significant overlap exists between GI and gynecologic causes of pain. This review outlines the most common of these disorders and includes some of the lesser common causes that, when missed, may result in poor patient outcomes.

ACUTE ABDOMINAL PAIN

Right Upper Quadrant

Acute cholecystitis

Definition: Acute inflammation of the gallbladder, usually as a result of obstruction of the cystic duct by a gallstone.

The obstruction of the cystic duct results in distension of the gallbladder, leading to visceral pain. The pain is typically described as a severe, steady ache, located predominantly in the right upper quadrant (RUQ) but can present with epigastrium. Radiation to the right subscapular area is common. Patients often report associated

Division of Gastroenterology and Hepatology, Saint Louis University, 3635 Vista Avenue, St Louis, MO 63110, USA

* Corresponding authors.

E-mail addresses: marsicanoe@gmail.com; pratherc@slu.edu

Obstet Gynecol Clin N Am 41 (2014) 465–489

http://dx.doi.org/10.1016/j.ogc.2014.06.002 obgyn.theclinics.com symptoms of nausea and vomiting. Most patients report having similar pain transiently in the past, especially after a meal high in fat.[1,2] This condition is known as biliary colic.

Providers should worry that their patient has developed acute cholecystitis when this pain has lasted greater than 4 to 6 hours and, especially, when associated with fever.

Symptoms

- RUQ pain
- Fever
- Nausea/vomiting (>50%)

Physical examination of the patient is useful, as diagnosis of acute cholecystitis is largely clinical and based on history. Findings of RUQ pain, fever, and leukocytosis strongly suggest acute cholecystitis. Jaundice, when present, suggests obstruction of the common bile duct either with a stone or from compression by the gallbladder (Mirizzi syndrome). A patient often has increased pain and inspiratory pause during palpation of the RUQ; this is known as Murphy sign. In 25% to 50% of patients, a large, distended gallbladder can also be palpated.[2]

Laboratory testing includes a complete blood count (CBC), assessment of liver chemistry (aspartate aminotransferase [AST], alanine aminotransferase [ALT], alkaline phosphatase, and total bilirubin), and determination of levels of amylase and lipase (both these to exclude coexistent pancreatitis). Mild elevations in the levels of serum bilirubin and alkaline phosphatase can be found in addition to an elevated white blood cell (WBC) count. Unlike cholangitis or common bile duct obstruction (choledocholithiasis), levels of AST and ALT are not commonly elevated.

Gallstones are demonstrated 90% to 95% on ultrasound (US) imaging in patients with acute cholecystitis; the additional findings of pericholecystic fluid, gallbladder wall thickening, and pain on compression of the gallbladder with the US probe (sonographic Murphy sign) are essentially diagnostic. A hepatobiliary iminodiacetic acid (HIDA) scan is rarely needed but can be used if the aforementioned workup is equivocal and there remains a high clinical suspicion or if acalculous cholecystitis is suspected. US imaging is preferred to computed tomographic (CT) scans, which more commonly miss the presence of gallstones. Further testing, including endoscopic US imaging, magnetic resonance cholangiopancreatography (MRCP), or endoscopic retrograde cholangiopancreatography (ERCP), are rarely necessary and reserved for when choledocholithiasis is suspected and not seen on other imaging procedures.[2,3]

Patients with acute cholecystitis should receive intravenous fluids, bowel rest, and symptomatic treatment of pain and nausea. When acute cholecystitis is confirmed, early surgical intervention (within 48–72 hours) remains the treatment of choice for patients with uncomplicated disease. Although debated in the past, early surgical intervention is preferred over delayed (after 6–8 weeks), as it decreases total length of hospitalization, morbidity, and mortality without increasing major risks of cholecystectomy.[4–6] If a patient's clinical condition does not allow surgical intervention, gallbladder drainage should be accomplished by endoscopic US-directed drainage, endoscopic placement of a drainage tube into the gallbladder via the cystic duct, or percutaneous drainage.

Broad-spectrum antibiotics are commonly given in acute cholecystitis. For suspected complicated cholecystitis, coverage with piperacillin/tazobactam, ampicillin/sulbactam, or a third-generation cephalosporin is used. Coverage of anaerobic organisms should be considered in sepsis and if gangrenous or emphysematous cholecystitis is suspected (along with urgent surgery or decompression).[2]

Complications of acute cholecystitis include emphysema, gangrene, perforation, fistulous formation (to duodenum, stomach, jejunum, colon, or abdominal wall), and gallstone ileus.

Differential diagnosis

- Abdominal aortic aneurysm
- Appendicitis
- Cholangiocarcinoma
- Cholangitis
- Choledocholithiasis
- Gallbladder cancer
- Gallbladder tumors
- Gastric ulcers
- Gastritis, acute
- Pancreatitis
- Pyelonephritis, acute

Acute cholecystitis in pregnancy is treated much the same with stabilization, antibiotics, and early surgical intervention. Typically fluoroquinolones and carbapenems are avoided because of concern for fetal toxicity.

Summary

Acute cholecystitis is a common cause of abdominal pain. It should be suspected in any patient with RUQ pain of greater than several hours, especially in those with fever and leukocytosis. US imaging is the best and most cost-effective imaging modality. Early surgical intervention, within 24 to 72 hours, decreases morbidity and mortality in most patients. Supportive measures include intravenous fluids, antibiotics, antiemetics, and pain control.

Acute cholangitis

Definition: Bile duct obstruction with superimposed infection of the biliary tree proximal to obstruction.

In the vast majority of cases, obstruction is the result of a stone; however, neoplasms, strictures, parasitic infections, and anatomic abnormalities can all result in cholangitis. High mortality rates exist in cholangitis; even with the advent of newer, noninvasive treatments, mortality remains as high as 30% in severe, acute cholangitis.[7]

The triad of RUQ pain, fever, and jaundice, known as the Charcot triad, is present in about 70% of patients.[8,9] The addition of mental status changes and shock to this triad is known as Reynolds pentad and is seen in severe cholangitis.[10] Some patients have minimal pain and present with chills and rigors. It should be noted that elderly or immunosuppressed patients can present atypically, with only mental status changes or sepsis.

Symptoms

- Fever and abdominal pain 80%
- Jaundice 60% to 70%

Laboratory studies typically reveal an elevated WBC count and abnormal liver chemistry (elevated alkaline phosphatase and ALT levels). The lipase level may also be elevated.[8,10]

The major imaging modalities of interest in cholangitis are abdominal US imaging and MRCP. US imaging identifies or infers the presence of a stone, by observing a dilated common bile duct, in up to 75% of cases.[11] If abdominal the US imaging result is negative but there is a high clinical suspicion, an MRCP should be ordered to further evaluate the biliary tree. The sensitivity and specificity of MRCP is comparable to that of ERCP in regards to detecting stones, sensitivity around 90% and specificity around 95%.[12]

When common bile duct stones are detected, ERCP should be urgently performed as a definitive treatment of the obstruction. Exact timing depends on the patient's clinical picture and may be subject to the availability of an advanced endoscopist. If an ERCP is unsuccessful, percutaneous transhepatic drainage can be accomplished by interventional radiology. In patients with failure to improve quickly with antibiotics, or whose clinical status declines, ERCP should be performed as soon as possible.

In suspected cholangitis, blood cultures should be taken and antibiotics initiated without delay. There is no consensus on the best empiric antibiotics for cholangitis. However, starting with a broad-spectrum antibiotic and narrowing based on culture is a reasonable option and includes the same choices as noted earlier for cholecystitis.

Summary

Cholangitis is an infection of the biliary tree resulting from obstruction, typically by a stone. Patients often complain of RUQ pain, fevers, rigors, and sometimes jaundice. If there is suspicion for cholangitis, basic laboratory tests and blood cultures should be drawn and broad-spectrum antibiotics started. Abdominal US imaging, or if needed MRCP, is used to locate the obstruction. ERCP is the treatment of choice, and timing of this procedure depends on the clinical status of the patient.

Budd-Chiari syndrome

Definition: Hepatic outflow obstruction, usually a result of thrombosis of the hepatic vein or suprahepatic inferior vena cava that results in sinusoidal congestion, portal vein hypertension, and reduced portal vein blood flow.

Budd-Chiari syndrome is most common in women in their third or fourth decades.[13] It can be the result of a myeloproliferative disorder, tumors, pregnancy, and other thrombogenic states, including cirrhosis. Risk factors are identified in more than 80% of patients.[14]

Clinical presentation can range from chronic symptoms to fulminant hepatic failure. Fulminant and acute Budd-Chiari syndromes most commonly occur in pregnant women, and typically, they had not previously been diagnosed with a prothrombotic condition.[15]

Signs and symptoms include abdominal pain, fever, hepatomegaly, jaundice, and new-onset ascites. Laboratory values for aminotransferases (ALT and AST) are often greater than 1000 units/L in fulminant disease, but in acute disease, they are usually 2 to 3 times the upper limit of normal. Acute disease may have a more indolent course; fulminant disease must be recognized, as it leads to rapid deterioration of the patient and carries a high mortality even with early detection and liver transplant.

Signs/symptoms

- Abdominal pain
- Fever
- Hepatomegaly
- Jaundice
- Ascites

Diagnosis is made by abdominal US imaging with Dopplers with a high sensitivity and specificity. CT or magnetic resonance imaging (MRI) with contrast is used as a confirmatory measure or if an experienced abdominal US imaging technician is not available.[14]

Treatment depends on the acuity, cause, and anatomic characteristics. A multidisciplinary approach is needed. Medical therapy with anticoagulation is aimed at the treatment of the sequelae of portal hypertension. Interventional radiology is used to decompress the portal venous system. Early transfer to a transplant center is recommended for patients with suspected fulminant Budd-Chiari syndrome.

Summary

Budd-Chiari syndrome results from hepatic outflow obstruction, most commonly from thrombosis. Clinically abdominal pain, hepatomegaly, jaundice, and elevated levels in liver function tests are found. Diagnosis is made using imaging, predominantly abdominal US imaging with Dopplers. Treatment depends on the acuity and cause of the disease and may include anticoagulation, radiologic decompression, or (in fulminant disease) liver transplant.

Hepatitis

Definition: Inflammation of the liver parenchyma.

Hepatitis is a general term that refers to a broad range of insults that lead to inflammation of the hepatic parenchyma. The most well-known are the acute hepatitides, hepatitis A, B, C, D, and E. Other viruses such as herpes, Epstein-Barr, cytomegalovirus, and even influenza can cause acute hepatitis. Other insults may be direct action of toxins/medications, autoimmune disorders, abnormal metabolism of copper/iron, and fatty deposition or other rare metabolic disorders.

Patients present with complaints of fatigue, RUQ abdominal pain, nausea, and anorexia. Elevated liver enzyme levels are noted on screening blood tests. An immediate viral hepatitis panel should be done. Autoimmune serologies and other specialized testing are ordered depending on the clinical situation and typically in consultation with a gastroenterologist/hepatologist. An abdominal US scan with Doppler of the hepatic vessels should be obtained to rule out biliary vascular causes.

Symptoms/signs
- Fatigue
- RUQ abdominal pain
- Nausea/vomiting
- Anorexia
- Jaundice

In pregnancy, particularly, hepatitis E is feared because of its progression to fulminant liver failure. Fatty liver of pregnancy most often occurs in the first trimester. The only treatment is prompt delivery of the fetus.[16]

Summary

Hepatitis, the inflammation of liver parenchyma, is caused by viruses, toxins, medications, autoimmune disorders, fatty deposition, and metabolic disorders, among others. Patients often present complaining of abdominal pain, nausea/vomiting, and fatigue. Evaluation should include blood work for the acute hepatitides and an abdominal US scan to rule out other causes of pathology.

Epigastric Pain

Perforated peptic ulcer

Definition: Perforation of the stomach or duodenum as a result of a peptic ulcer.

Peptic ulcer disease (PUD) is common and refers to both gastric and duodenal ulcers (DUs). The most common causes include *Helicobacter pylori* infection or nonsteroidal antiinflammatory drug (NSAID) use. Although the morbidity and mortality from PUD has declined in the last century, perforation remains a serious complication with high mortality.[8,17]

Peptic ulcer perforation presents clinically as peritonitis without defining features, rebound, guarding, and diffuse abdominal pain. If the patient is able, however, a history of PUD, recent NSAID use, chronic use of antacid medications, or evidence of upper GI bleeding may increase suspicion. Many patients presenting with perforation have no preceding chronic abdominal pain.

Signs/symptoms

- Rebound
- Guarding
- Peritonitis
- Crepitus

There may be free air found under the diaphragm in abdominal radiographs, but a CT scan can usually establish a diagnosis.[18]

Cornerstone of treatment includes stabilization, intravenous proton pump inhibitors (PPIs), broad spectrum antibiotics, and emergent surgical intervention.[8]

Summary

PUD is common and refers to ulcers in both the stomach and the duodenum. Perforation of one of these ulcers results in acute abdominal pain and peritonitis. Diagnosis can usually be established using a CT scan. Timely evaluation, antibiotics, and surgical intervention are needed.

Acute pancreatitis

Definition: Acute pancreatitis is an acute inflammatory disorder of the pancreas with involvement of the peripancreatic tissues and possibly other organ systems.

Acute pancreatitis is one of the most common inpatient GI diagnoses in the United States and is a source of significant morbidity and mortality.[19] Although gallstones and alcohol are the most common causes of pancreatitis in the United States, other considerations such as autoimmune disorders, drugs, smoking, hypercalcemia, hypertriglyceridemia, and genetic predisposition must be considered. Acute pancreatitis can occur in patients with acute fatty liver of pregnancy and should be suspected with abdominal pain or nausea and vomiting. Around 25% of cases of pancreatitis remain idiopathic after a thorough workup.[20] **Table 1** presents the causes of acute pancreatitis.

Table 1
Causes of acute pancreatitis

Causes of Acute Pancreatitis	Some Common Medications Associated with Acute Pancreatitis
Alcohol	Thiazide diuretics
Cholelithiasis	Furosemide
Drugs	Sulfonamides
Hypertriglyceridemia	Azathioprine
Infections, ie, mumps	Tetracyclines
Trauma	Valproic acid
Pancreas divisum	Estrogens

Adapted from Feldman M, Friedman L. Sleisenger and Fordtran's gastrointestinal and liver disease. Philadelphia: Saunders (Elsevier); 2010; with permission.

Clinically, most patients complain of abdominal pain, usually located in the epigastrium, but the pain may present in the RUQ or the left upper quadrant (LUQ).[21] Radiation through to the back occurs in approximately half of patients. Most patients report nausea and vomiting at presentation.[22–24] Elevations in amylase or lipase levels greater than 3 times the upper limit of normal, in the absence of renal failure, are typically found in acute pancreatitis.[20] WBC count is frequently elevated, as are the hemoglobin/hematocrit levels as a function of hemoconcentration. Elevations in the levels of transaminase can be seen, especially in gallstone pancreatitis.

Physical examination findings vary depending on the severity of pancreatitis. Patients with mild symptoms could exhibit minimal tenderness, whereas those with severe disease can have significant pain on palpation. Hypoactive bowel sounds and abdominal distension are seen in cases of ileus secondary to inflammation. Scleral icterus may be observed in the presence of obstructive jaundice. Those patients with severe pancreatitis have signs and symptoms that reflect the presence of systemic inflammatory response syndrome (SIRS), such as fever, tachypnea, tachycardia, and elevated WBC count. Decreased breath sounds in the lung bases secondary to pleural effusions are possible. Cullen sign (periumbilical ecchymosis) and Grey Turner sign (flank ecchymosis) are rare but can be seen in hemorrhagic pancreatitis. **Table 2** lists the symptoms, signs, and laboratory tests associated with acute pancreatitis.[20]

Diagnosis of pancreatitis is made when 2 of 3 of the following criteria are met[1]: acute onset of persistent, severe, epigastric pain often radiating to the back[2]; elevation in serum lipase or amylase level to 3 times or greater than the upper limit of normal[3]; and characteristic findings of acute pancreatitis on imaging.[22] In patients with classic abdominal pain and elevations in amylase or lipase level, imaging is not needed to confirm diagnosis. However, abdominal US scan should be obtained to rule out biliary pathology.

CT with contrast is the imaging modality of choice if a confirmation of diagnosis is needed.[20] MRI and MRCP can also be used to evaluate the biliary tree for pathology.

Severity of pancreatitis should be established in every patient. Several scores exist to prognosticate outcomes of patients; the score most commonly used at present is the bedside index of severity in acute pancreatitis (BISAP), which is assessed in the first 24 hours (1 point each for blood urea nitrogen >25, impaired mental status, ≥2 SIRS criteria, age >60 years, presence of pleural effusion). Mortality increases greatly with a score of 3 or more and a mortality of 22% when all criteria are present. Those patients with predicted or actual severe disease should be triaged to an intensive care unit (ICU).

Table 2
Symptoms, signs, and laboratory tests associated with acute pancreatitis

Symptoms	Signs	Laboratory Tests
Epigastric/RUQ abdominal pain	Epigastric tenderness	Elevations in amylase and/or lipase levels
Bandlike radiation of pain to back	Hypoactive bowel sounds	Elevated WBC count
Nausea and/or vomiting	Icterus	Elevated hemoglobin/ hematocrit levels
	Fever, tachycardia, tachypnea	Elevations in liver function test values (gallstone)
	Cullen sign	
	Grey Turner sign	

Data from Forsmark CE, Baillie J, AGA Institute Clinical Practice and Economics Committee, AGA Institute Governing Board. AGA Institute technical review on acute pancreatitis. Gastroenterology 2007;132(5):2022–44.

Initial treatment considerations for all patients include aggressive fluid resuscitation with lactated Ringer solutions, pain control, and bowel rest. In those patients who are likely not to be given oral foods for greater than 7 days, a nasojejunal tube should be placed for enteral feedings with a semielemental formula.[20,21] Patients with diagnosed gallstone pancreatitis should undergo ERCP if there is suspicion for a retained common bile duct stone. These patients should also undergo cholecystectomy once they have recovered.[20] There is no role for prophylactic antibiotics in mild or severe pancreatitis. Patients with suspected sepsis should be given broad-spectrum antibiotics until they are confirmed culture negative.[25]

Superinfection of pancreatic necrosis usually does not present before 7 to 10 days. If it is suspected, an effort to obtain tissues should be made; however, antibiotic use can also be started in the absence of tissue diagnosis. There is not a consensus in the literature about the correct management. Either way, if a patient becomes clinically unstable, surgical intervention should be considered. If a patient remains stable, debridement should be delayed at least 4 weeks and reassessed at that time.[25]

Summary

Acute pancreatitis is an acute inflammatory disorder of the pancreas, often a result of gallstones or alcohol. It is diagnosed by meeting 2 of the following 3 criteria[1]: acute onset of persistent, severe, epigastric pain often radiating to the back[2]; elevation in serum lipase or amylase levels to 3 times or greater than the upper limit of normal[3]; and characteristic findings of acute pancreatitis on imaging. Abdominal US scan should be obtained to ensure that biliary stones are retained in the common bile duct, and if so, an ERCP should be performed. CT with contrast is a useful mode of imaging, either to augment diagnosis or after 72 hours to evaluate the extent of necrosis. Early evaluation of the severity of pancreatitis should be made. Mainstays of therapy include aggressive fluid resuscitation and pain control. Antibiotics are rarely necessary in acute pancreatitis in the absence of sepsis.

Right Lower Quadrant

Acute appendicitis

Definition: Inflammation of the vestigial vermiform appendix.

Appendicitis is one of the most common acute abdominal complaints in the United States and the leading cause of emergent abdominal surgeries in the world.[19,26] It is most commonly found in the second and third decades, with a male predominance.[26]

The classic presentation is described as mild periumbilical abdominal pain migrating to the right lower quadrant (RLQ) and increasing in intensity, eventually associated with nausea, vomiting, and anorexia, which is seen in up to 60% of patients.[8] Other features that may be atypical or nonspecific include indigestion, flatulence, diarrhea, bowel irregularity, and general malaise.[27]

On physical examination, patients may have a low-grade temperature. Fever, when noted, is usually later in the course and is low grade in the absence appendiceal perforation and peritonitis.[28] Patients tend to lie still and have RLQ abdominal tenderness with some degree of guarding. Rebound, if found in the RLQ, is a sensitive predictor.[27] Other findings include the following:

- Rovsing sign → pain in the RLQ with palpation of the left lower quadrant (LLQ)
- Psoas sign → RLQ pain with passive extension of right hip
- Obturator sign → RLQ pain with passive flexion of the right hip and knee followed by internal rotation of the right hip

The above-mentioned findings depend on the location of the appendix, which can differ between patients.

Laboratory studies are of limited use. Most patients have a mild leukocytosis.[28]

Abdominal imaging should not be relied on heavily, as a classic history, physical, and laboratory examination can be diagnostic in up to 90% of cases.[29] However, if the diagnosis remains unclear, imaging is a useful adjunct. CT with contrast is preferred, unless the patient is pregnant, and then an abdominal US scan is the study of choice.

The gold standard in the treatment of appendicitis remains surgical. Occasionally pain medication and antibiotics are used if a surgeon is not readily available.

Diagnostic challenges

Appendicitis in pregnancy Diagnosis of appendicitis in pregnancy is a challenge, particularly because the appendix is displaced cephalad as the uterus grows (**Fig. 1**). Otherwise, many of the symptoms of nausea, vomiting, and anorexia are similar, but the cause of these symptoms becomes blurred in pregnancy.[30] The incidence of fetal loss increases substantially in perforated appendicitis; therefore, early diagnosis is important. An abdominal US scan is often needed because of an atypical history, but it should not be relied on, as the sensitivity and specificity are low. CT imaging can be obtained in cases of inconclusive US imaging and has been shown to decrease the negative appendectomy rate, but the risk of radiation must be considered.[7]

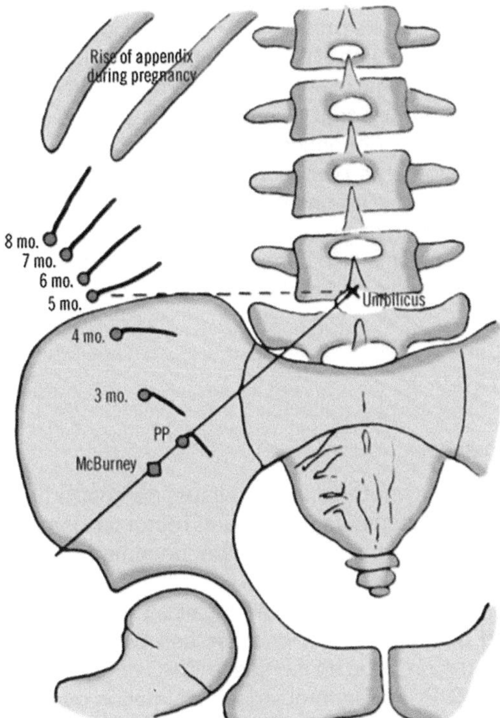

Fig. 1. Location of appendix in pregnant woman based on gestation. (*From* Skandalakis JE, Colborn GL. Skandalakis' surgical anatomy: the embryologic and anatomic basis of modern surgery. Athens (Greece): Paschalidis Medical Publications Ltd; 2004; with permission.)

Atypical appendicitis A retrocecal (ileal) appendicitis often presents with less pain due to shielding by the abdominal wall. Pelvic appendicitis may be associated with fecal and urinary urgency. A high level of suspicion and CT scan are necessary for diagnosis.[8]

Summary

Acute appendicitis is the most common surgical abdominal emergency in the United States. It is a result of inflammation of the vestigial vermiform appendix, usually secondary to obstruction or infection. The classic clinical history is of epigastric pain increasing and migrating to the RLQ, associated with nausea, vomiting, and anorexia. In pregnancy, the appendix is displaced, causing an atypical presentation; therefore, a clinician must have high suspicion. Physical examination is consistent with local peritonitis. The vast majority of patients can be diagnosed clinically; however, if imaging is required to confirm, the test of choice is CT scan.

Left Upper Quadrant

The most common causes of LUQ abdominal pain include PUD (discussed elsewhere)[31–34] and gastritis (discussed elsewhere).[35,36] Less common causes include splenic abscess, splenic infarct or rupture, and subdiaphragmatic abscesses.

Left Lower Quadrant

Colonic diverticulitis

Definition: Inflammation of a diverticulum within the colon.

Diverticula are acquired saclike protrusions from the colonic wall, involving the mucosa and submucosa. Inflammation of these diverticula is known as diverticulitis and occurs in 10% to 25% of people with diverticula.[31] Men and women are equally affected.[32]

Diverticulitis should be considered in patients who present with lower abdominal pain, fever, and leukocytosis. Abdominal pain is often present in the LLQ, although, based on individual anatomy and location of the inflamed diverticulum, it can also be suprapubic or right sided. The onset of this pain is insidious, over several days before presentation. It is often associated with changes in bowel habits, but bleeding is rarely reported. Many patients also complain of some nausea and vomiting. Urinary symptoms, when present, indicate irritation of the bladder wall.[33]

Signs/symptoms

- Abdominal pain
- Fever
- Leukocytosis
- Radiographic findings

Less common signs or symptoms include ileus, peritonitis (if the inflammation is no longer localized), colocutaneous fistula, and rectal tenderness (with a low-lying pelvic abscess). Hypotension and shock are uncommon unless there is frank perforation.[33]

On physical examination, there is typically localized tenderness in the LLQ, with or without rebound and guarding. A tender mass can be palpated in around 20% of patients.[31] Fever is common, as is an increased WBC count or inflammatory markers (eg, C-reactive protein [CRP] or erythrocyte sedimentation rate [ESR]).

Diverticulitis is classified as uncomplicated or complicated. Uncomplicated diverticulitis is the result of a localized phlegmon, whereas complicated diverticulitis is associated with abscess, free perforation, fistula, or obstruction.[2] **Box 1** details the surgical staging of diverticultis.[2]

Box 1
Surgical staging of diverticulitis

Stage 1—Confined pericolic abscess

Stage 2—Distant abscess

Stage 3—Purulent peritonitis

Stage 4—Fecal peritonitis

Adapted from Feldman M, Friedman L. Sleisenger and Fordtran's gastrointestinal and liver disease. Philadelphia: Saunders (Elsevier); 2010; with permission.

Antibiotic therapy, aimed against gram-negative rods and anaerobes, should be initiated orally, as an outpatient, or intravenously, as an inpatient, depending on the severity of illness.[34] Antibiotic coverage is broadened in patients who require ICU-level care. Those patients who present with diffuse peritonitis or who fail medical therapy and/or percutaneous drainage should be considered for surgery.[35]

Summary

Diverticulitis is the inflammation of saclike protrusions from the colonic wall, involving the mucosa and submucosa. Diagnosis is made using clinical history coupled with laboratory and imaging data (abdominal pain, fever, leukocytosis, and radiographic findings). Antibiotics should be given to all patients diagnosed with diverticulitis; the choice of antibiotic is based on the severity of illness. Surgical intervention is reserved for fulminant disease or for those who have failed medical therapy.

Diffuse

Acute mesenteric ischemia

Definition: Acute mesenteric ischemia (AMI) is the result of decreased intestinal blood flow, either venous or arterial, typically as a result of occlusion, hypoperfusion, or vasospasm.

Clinicians should be highly suspicious in the following cases:

- Elderly patients with acute onset of severe abdominal pain and history of vasculopathy
- Patients with cardiac arrhythmias or known prothrombotic states
- Pain out of proportion to examination

AMI can be difficult to diagnose and carries high morbidity and mortality rates, especially when the diagnosis is delayed. Most commonly, ischemia is the result of arterial occlusion (85%–95%), with venous occlusion accounting for around 5% and nonocclusive ischemia 15%.[36]

A careful history can reveal personal or family history of an embolic event or thrombosis. Antecedent symptoms of chronic mesenteric ischemia (weight loss, postprandial abdominal pain, and sitophobia) are not uncommon in mesenteric arterial occlusion.

Suspicion should be increased in patients who are older than 50 years, in cardiac patients (congestive heart failure, recent myocardial infarction, and arrhythmia), or in patients with other known vascular disease who present with severe, acute abdominal pain. The pain is classically described as being out of proportion to the physical examination. Especially at the onset, the abdomen is flat, soft, and nontender. The pain can be followed by a sudden, forceful bowel movement. Nausea and vomiting are also common.[37]

Later in the course, peritoneal signs become evident as the bowel becomes infarcted, leading to gangrene and possible perforation. Abdominal distension, absence of bowel sounds, mental status changes, elevations in the WBC count and amylase levels, and lactic acidosis are found later in the disease process as well and portend a bad outcome.

Signs/symptoms

- Abdominal pain is out of proportion to examination
- Nausea/vomiting
- Peritoneal signs later in the course

Diagnosis of AMI relies on imaging. Per American Gastroenterology Association guidelines, patients suspected of having AMI should have a prompt CT angiography. Findings include bowel wall thickening, lack of arterial enhancement, arterial occlusion, venous thrombosis, engorgement of mesenteric veins, intramural gas, and mesenteric or portal gas. If the CT angiography is suggestive, a prompt selective angiogram should be performed, and it remains the gold standard of diagnosis, with a sensitivity and specificity approaching 100%.[37]

Successful treatment depends on early diagnosis of AMI, with early reperfusion. If it is not made before intestinal infarction, mortality rate approaches 70% to 90%.[38] Broad-spectrum antibiotics should be given. Once the lesion is identified, the patient is vascularized surgically or endovascularly. Papaverine, a phosphodiesterase inhibitor, is also used preoperatively and postoperatively for vasodilation. Patients with peritoneal signs or suspicion of perforation usually are headed directly to surgery.[37]

Special consideration Mesenteric venous thrombosis, although rare, should also be considered in patients with acute abdominal pain, as the presentation is similar. History is important, as a hypercoagulable condition can be identified in most of these patients.[39] Diagnosis is made with contrast CT in the vast majority of cases; however, selective angiography remains the gold standard. Treatment of symptomatic, acute venous thrombosis mimics that of arterial occlusion as described earlier. If the patient is asymptomatic, they are often given anticoagulants for 6 months and reassessed.[37]

Summary

AMI is the result of decreased intestinal blood flow, either venous or arterial, typically as a result of occlusion, hypoperfusion, or vasospasm.

AMI should be considered early in patients who present with acute abdominal pain out of proportion to examination, especially if they are elders, have an arrhythmia, or have a history of vasculopathy. Delayed diagnosis can lead to extremely high mortality rates. CT angiography is typically the first imaging test of choice and has good sensitivity and specificity. Selective angiography remains the gold standard in diagnosis and can also contribute therapeutically. Relief of the obstruction either surgically or endovascularly should be performed emergently.

Bowel obstruction

Definition: Impairment of normal flow through the small bowel, either by mechanical means or secondary to abnormal motility (ileus).

Although not all bowel obstructions require surgical intervention, they remain a common surgical emergency and account for around 300,000 laparotomies a year. The most common cause, which accounts for more than half of obstructions, is adhesions. Abdominal wall hernias and neoplasms are also common considerations.[40] Less commonly found are volvulus, intra-abdominal abscesses, inflammatory strictures, gallstones, parasites, among others. **Box 2** lists the causes of bowel obstruction.

Patients classically present with acute onset of abdominal pain, nausea, vomiting, and progressive abdominal distension, obstipation and abdominal distension being the most common.[41] Symptoms vary based on the degree, site, duration, and cause of obstruction. Blood tests may reveal leukocytosis, electrolyte abnormalities, or acidosis.

Symptoms/signs

- Abdominal pain
- Nausea/vomiting
- Progressive abdominal distension
- Obstipation

Suspicion of a small-bowel obstruction (SBO) is confirmed radiologically. Initial evaluation with an abdominal radiograph (both upright and lateral decubitus) is both quick and inexpensive and therefore a good option for initial imaging. Dilated loops of bowel with air fluid levels can confirm a SBO (**Fig. 2**). However, a CT scan with intravenous contrast (oral if patient can tolerate) is better at delineating the specific site of obstruction, cause, as well as having improved sensitivity and specificity for diagnosis.[41] As a result, CT scans should be ordered when the diagnosis is unclear after abdominal radiography, to identify the specific site of obstruction or to evaluate the cause (ie, hernia, mass). Proximal obstructions may not present with an abundance of air fluid levels.

Initial management includes hydration, correction of any metabolic abnormalities, placement of nasogastric tube for decompression, and bowel rest. Around 64% to 73% of patients can be managed successfully conservatively.[42] Those who fail conservative management or clinically deteriorate require surgical intervention with either open or laparoscopic surgery, both of which have decreased morbidity and mortality in recent years.

Summary

Bowel obstruction is the result of impairment of normal flow through the small bowel, by mechanical means or secondary to abnormal motility (ileus). The most common cause is adhesions, although hernias and neoplasms are often the culprit. Basic blood work should be obtained; however, diagnosis is made radiologically with abdominal plain films and CT scans. Medical management is often successful, but for those patients who fail or worsen clinically, definitive treatment is surgical.

Box 2
Causes of small-bowel obstruction

Abdominal wall hernias

Volvulus

Inflammatory strictures

Parasites

Neoplasms

Intra-abdominal abscesses

Gallstones

Data from Miller G, Boman J, Shrier I, et al. Etiology of small bowel obstruction. Am J Surg 2000;180(1):33–6.

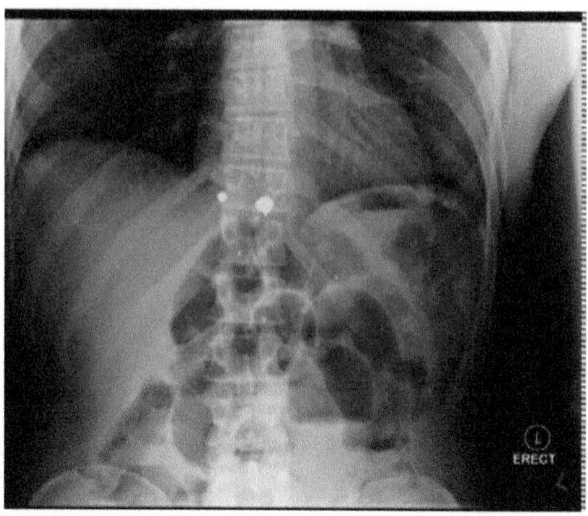

Fig. 2. Abdominal radiograph showing dilated loops of small bowel with air fluid levels consistent with small bowel obstruction.

CHRONIC ABDOMINAL PAIN SYNDROMES

Right Upper Quadrant

Biliary colic

Definition: An intense, dull discomfort located in the RUQ or epigastrium that may radiate to the back (including the right shoulder blade).

Despite the name, biliary colic is not colicky. History may reveal recurrent, moderate to severe, dull, or a boring RUQ or epigastrium pain that may or may not radiate to the back or right scapular region, occurring typically within hours of a meal, lasting at least 30 minutes, plateauing within an hour, and subsiding within 6 hours. The pain may localize to the RUQ if the gallbladder irritates the peritoneum; thus, patients may reposition themselves for comfort. About 10% to 25% of patients with gallstones become symptomatic during a 10-year period. Twenty percent of patients with biliary colic develop acute cholecystitis. Because it is often a precursor event, biliary colic falls within the same spectrum of biliary tract disease as cholecystitis, choledocholithiasis, and cholangitis.[43]

Signs/symptoms

- Constant abdominal pain
- Precipitated by fatty meals
- Frequently occurs at night

Risk factors include female sex, pregnancy, and rapid weight loss. Diagnosis is confirmed preferentially by US imaging, with CT scans missing 20% of stones. Treatment of biliary colic with confirmed gallstones is laparoscopic cholecystectomy because of its high success rate and low risk of complications. Oral dissolution therapy with bile acids can be considered with cholesterol stones less than 5 mm in diameter, although the stones recur when the therapy is stopped. While patients are waiting for surgery, a low-fat diet is prudent.

Epigastric

Peptic ulcer disease

Definition: PUD is the disruption of the mucosal integrity of the stomach, duodenum, or both, caused by local inflammation, leading to a well-defined mucosal defect.

PUD includes gastric ulcers (GUs) and DUs. It can present acutely as previously mentioned in the form of bleeding, perforation, or obstruction. However, it commonly is the cause of chronic epigastric pain. The epigastric pain can be a burning or gnawing discomfort or "hunger pain," although the symptoms are not specific to GU or DU. DU pain typically occurs 1 to 3 hours after a meal and may improve with food or antacids. It is not infrequent for patients to have pain shortly after bedtime (midnight to 3 AM), which may awaken them from sleep. GU pain typically is exacerbated by food and may also be more accompanied by nausea and weight loss. PUD can also commonly have dyspeptic symptoms: early satiety, postprandial nausea, or belching.[44,45]

Differential diagnosis

- Cholecystitis
- Cholangitis
- Gastroenteritis
- Functional (nonulcer) dyspepsia
- Inflammatory bowel disease (IBD)
- Acute coronary syndrome
- Abdominal aortic aneurysm
- Acute hepatitis of various causes

Most cases of PUD are related to NSAID use or *H pylori* infection. In addition, common risk factors include a prior history of PUD, NSAID use, and smoking. A diagnosis of PUD is obtained via upper endoscopic evaluation demonstrating the presence of ulceration. A diagnosis of PUD can be inferred in low-risk patients not previously investigated with *H pylori* testing (typically the stool antigen test) and treatment initiated. Upper endoscopy is indicated when patients present with nonspecific symptoms of dyspepsia in the setting of alarm symptoms such as bleeding or anemia, early satiety, weight loss, dysphagia or odynophagia, recurrent emesis, middle-aged patients (>45–50 years), and family history of upper GI tract malignancy. Most patients with dyspeptic symptoms do not have ulcers but have functional dyspepsia (or may have gallstones).[46]

Once the diagnosis is established, the history of NSAID use should be reviewed and also test for *H pylori* should be obtained; this can be achieved with gastric biopsies at endoscopy (via a rapid urease test), fecal stool antigen test, or the more expensive urea breath testing. In addition, if there are multiple ulcers or large or giant ulcers, then testing for Zollinger-Ellison syndrome should be entertained by checking a serum fasting gastrin level.

Cessation of NSAIDs is essential in NSAID-induced PUD, if feasible. If not, then concurrent use of a PPI or prostaglandin analogue has been shown to reduce the risk of recurrence.[47]

Patients who test positive for *H pylori* should be treated with a triple-therapy regimen. In patients with complicated PUD (bleeding, perforation, and obstruction), *H pylori* eradication should be confirmed via follow-up stool antigen testing.

Patients with GUs should undergo repeat upper endoscopic evaluation in 6 to 8 weeks to document healing, as opposed to those with DUs who do not require follow-up endoscopy, unless the ulcers are giant (larger than 2 cm in size).

Maintenance antisecretory therapy should be considered after *H pylori* is eradicated or the documented ulcer has healed in high-risk subgroups such as those who require long-term anticoagulation, history of complicated PUD, refractory or giant ulcers.[48] See **Fig. 3** for a picture of a GU.

Summary

PUD includes gastric and/or DUs. Symptoms include chronic epigastric pain that may be worse after meals or at night (DUs). Alarm symptoms such as bleeding or anemia, early satiety, weight loss, dysphagia or odynophagia, recurrent emesis, or presentation in middle-aged patients (45–50 years) or older may warrant endoscopic evaluation. *H pylori* testing should be obtained if PUD is confirmed. Treatment includes cessation of NSAIDs for NSAID-induced PUD and treatment of *H pylori* infection if testing result is positive. Eradication of *H pylori* is warranted in complicated PUD cases. Maintenance antisecretory therapy should be considered in high-risk subgroups.

Gastritis

Definition: Inflammation-associated mucosal injury to the stomach.

Gastritis is often secondary to infections (*H pylori*), exogenous irritants (NSAIDs, alcohol—more correctly termed gastropathy), autoimmunity, or less frequently ischemia.

Symptoms are often vague and nonspecific. Patients may complain of epigastric pain, and thus it should be considered in the differential of dyspepsia. Discomfort has typically been present for several weeks to months leading up to presentation. Review of medications for offending agents and social history of alcohol use are important when taking a history. Examination often reveals some epigastric tenderness.

Diagnosis is made by visualization with endoscopy and biopsy of the gastric tissue. Endoscopically the mucosa is found to be erythematous with or without superficial erosions (**Fig. 4**). Erythema may be patchy or diffuse.[49] Adjunctive biochemical testing that can help include serologic testing for *H pylori* or evaluation of antibodies for autoimmune gastritis.[50]

Treatment is determined by the cause of the gastritis. Treatment of *H pylori* is required if found. Discontinuation of offending agents such as NSAIDs or alcohol can also be recommended. PPIs or histamine 2 receptor blockers are also used adjunctively to help heal the mucosa.

Summary

Gastritis, inflammation of stomach tissue, is defined on biopsy via endoscopy. It can have many causes, including infections, autoimmunity, exogenous irritants, and ischemia. Patients often complain of long-standing dyspepsia, and a careful social and medication history should be taken. Adjunctive testing including serologic testing for *H pylori* and autoimmune serologies can be useful in specific patients. Treatment depends on the cause of gastritis; however, PPIs and H2 blockers are often used adjunctively.

Functional dyspepsia

Definition: Defined by the presence of epigastric pain/burning, early satiety, and fullness with no evidence of organic disease to explain the symptoms. Symptoms should persist for at least 3 to 6 months.

Just as in irritable bowel syndrome (IBS), visceral hypersensitivity, altered gut microbiota, and psychosocial dysfunction are believed to play a large role in functional dyspepsia.[51]

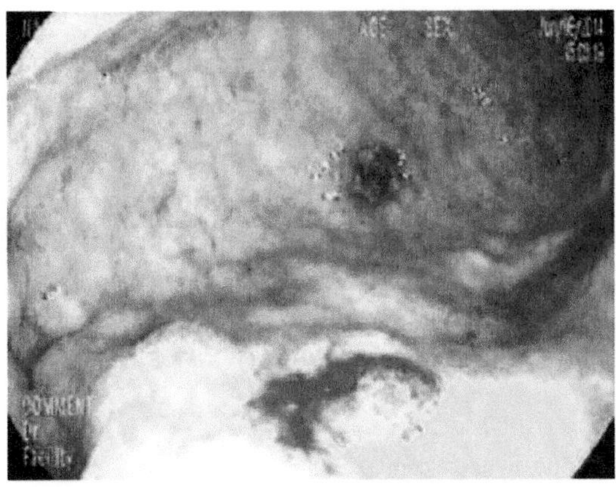

Fig. 3. Clean based gastric ulcer.

Symptoms

- Abdominal pain, especially in the epigastrium
- Abdominal burning
- Bloating
- Postprandial fullness
- Early satiety
- Nausea

A diagnosis of functional dyspepsia is typically made after the exclusion of other causes of dyspepsia (as outlined previously in this article), including upper endoscopy. See **Box 3** for differential diagnosis.

Initial treatment approach usually includes a trial of PPIs for 6 to 8 weeks. Tricyclic antidepressents are a good second-line approach, in hopes to alleviate pain via neuromodulation. Promotility agents are useful in people suspected to have a component of delayed gastric emptying. In patients with significant amounts of pain and

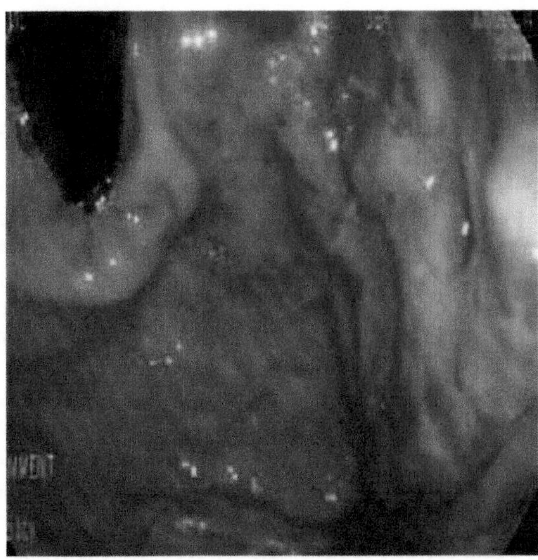

Fig. 4. Gastritis.

Box 3
Differential diagnosis of functional dyspepsia

Peptic ulcer disease

Gastroesophageal reflux disease

Biliary cholic

Gastroparesis

Chronic pancreatitis

Abdominal wall pain

Gastric carcinoma

Infiltrative diseases (ie, sarcoid)

Metabolic disturbances (ie, hypercalcemia)

Medications

Data from Greenberger N, Blumberg RS, Burakoff R. Current diagnosis and treatment: gastroenterology, hepatology, and endoscopy. New York: McGraw-Hill; 2009.

bloating, peppermint oil has been shown to be of benefit. Psychological therapy for those with psychiatric comorbidities is also appropriate.[52]

Summary

Functional dyspepsia is defined by the presence of epigastric pain/burning, early satiety, fullness without evidence of organic disease for a period of at least 3 to 6 months. Diagnosis is usually made after a thorough evaluation rules out alternative diagnosis and should include an upper endoscopy. Treatment with a PPI should be initiated first, followed by a trial of tricyclic antidepressants if PPI fails. Alternative therapies including treatment of psychological comorbidities should also be entertained.

Chronic pancreatitis

Definition: Chronic inflammation of the pancreas leading to permanent structural damage and the development of exocrine and endocrine insufficiency.

The diagnosis of chronic pancreatitis is difficult to ascertain, especially in its early stages. Known risk factors include alcohol, smoking, ductal abnormalities, autoimmunity, and genetic (familial) factors.

The classic clinical description is of pain and pancreatic insufficiency, usually in the form of diarrhea or malabsorption. However, this is only in the end stages of the disease. Early in the course of chronic pancreatitis, pain is often the only symptom.

The abdominal pain is typically epigastric and often radiates to the back. It can often be intermittent at the beginning and progresses to constant pain over time. The pain is often difficult to treat.[53] Although pain is a dominant feature, up to 20% of people with evidence of exocrine pancreatic insufficiency report no pain.[54]

Pancreatic insufficiency can come in the form of endocrine insufficiency, that is, diabetes, or exocrine insufficiency manifesting as diarrhea and fat-soluble vitamin malabsorption. Weight loss because of fat malabsorption occurs late in the disease process.

Diagnosis is challenging and includes laboratory studies, imaging studies, and endoscopic evaluation with endoscopic ultrasound (EUS) and possible biopsy.

Useful laboratory tests include fecal elastase, stool qualitative fat (and sometimes quantitative fat), autoimmune serologies, IgG-4, and A1c. Genetic testing can also be done when appropriate (eg, cystic fibrosis transmembrane conductance regulator [CFTR], protease, serine, 1 (trypsin 1) [PRSS]).

Imaging studies including radiography, CT, and MRI are useful. A radiograph that reveals calcifications in the pancreas is diagnostic but rarely seen. CT and MRI are good at evaluating the parenchyma and pancreatic duct abnormalities that are often seen in chronic pancreatitis.[55]

EUS is becoming more widely available and has been found to be sensitive and specific, especially in the setting of early disease that is difficult to diagnose. Certain diagnostic criterion has been developed specifically using EUS.[56] If needed, a biopsy can also be done during this procedure to evaluate for autoimmune pancreatitis or carcinoma.

Differential diagnosis is broad and can consist of PUD, IBS/functional abdominal pain, and IBD.

It is a difficult disorder to diagnose because of the chronic pain syndrome that is associated with it, as well as the absence of easily obtainable objective evidence to support the diagnosis.

Treatment begins with lifestyle modifications, including cessation of alcohol and smoking. Patients are encouraged to eat frequent, low-fat meals. Pain management becomes the cornerstone of treatment in most patients with a strong preference for avoiding narcotics if at all possible. Pancreatic enzyme supplementation is useful in some patients. Those with obstruction of the pancreatic duct should undergo ERCP to attempt decompression. Neuromodulation with tricylic antidepressants is used with some success. Long-term, severe pain ultimately requires narcotics. Procedures such as celiac plexus block can relieve pain but have not provided long-term benefit for most patients.[56,57] In extreme cases, surgery can be contemplated but is most successful when there is clear evidence of pancreatic duct obstruction.

Summary

Chronic pancreatitis is the end result of long-term inflammation in the pancreas leading to endocrine/exocrine insufficiency and pain in most patients. Patients present with epigastric pain, either intermittent or constant; diarrhea; fat-soluble vitamin deficiencies; and diabetes. Diagnosis is difficult, but clinical suspicion along with laboratory testing, imaging, and procedures can be revealing. Treatment primarily targets pain, after lifestyle modifications are made. Pancreatic enzyme replacement, neuromodulation, and, sometimes, narcotics are cornerstones of therapy.

RLQ PAIN

Hernias

Inflammatory bowel disease

Definition: Chronic inflammation of the GI tract.

IBD comprises 2 diseases, Crohn disease (CD) and ulcerative colitis (UC). Of the two, CD is most likely to present with abdominal pain. Although pain is present in UC, rectal bleeding and diarrhea are the predominant symptoms. It is thought that immune dysregulation, genetic susceptibilities, and fecal microbiota are related to disease susceptibility in the IBDs.[8]

In UC, inflammation is limited to the mucosal layer of the colon. Inflammation characteristically begins in the rectum and extends proximally to encompass part or all of the large intestine. Patients present with rectal bleeding and tenesmus, and depending on the extent of inflammation, abdominal pain and diarrhea may also be major issues. Because UC is noted to improve with smoking, often patients come for initial presentation after they have recently quit. A recent history of smoking cessation increases the likelihood that these symptoms are due to UC. During physical examination, abdominal tenderness, particularly in the LLQ, can be noted. Rectal examination can reveal bloody stool. Although most patients are managed medically, total colectomy is curative for patients with UC.[3,8]

Inflammation in CD is transmural, which accounts for many of the complications, including fistulas, abscesses, and strictures. Unlike in UC, the inflammation in CD can be in any area of the alimentary tract, most often in the terminal ileum and cecum. Patients typically complain of abdominal pain, diarrhea, weight loss, and bloody stools (although rectal bleeding is less frequent than in UC). Bowel obstruction is not uncommon in stricturing disease. Patients can present with perianal disease, including fissures and perianal fistula, in the absence of other colonic symptoms. Unlike UC, smoking worsens CD, and patients should be counseled as such. Symptoms from complications can also be seen on presentation.

Extraintestinal manifestations can be found in both CD and UC and can involve but are not limited to arthritis (common), eye involvement, skin disorders, pulmonary involvement, renal stones, and vitamin deficiencies.

Physical examination can note abdominal tenderness, classically in the RLQ. Malnutrition can be seen, especially in those with significant small-bowel inflammation.[8,58,59]

Diagnosis is made by careful history, physical examination, and laboratory, radiographic, endoscopic, and pathologic findings. Helpful laboratory findings include stool studies for infection and inflammatory markers (eg, calprotectin and/or lactoferrin), inflammatory markers in the serum (eg, CRP or ESR), CBC, iron studies, vitamin B12 (in CD), and chemistry panel (especially low albumin levels). Imaging studies such as CT are useful at evaluating for strictures, abscesses, or masses. With the advent of CT or MRI enterography, much better evaluation can be made of the small bowel. Capsule endoscopy can also be used to evaluate parts of the small bowel that cannot be seen endoscopically.[8,58] Autoimmune markers, including anti-saccharomyces cerevisiae antibody (ASCA) and perinuclear anti-neutrophil cytoplasmic antibody (p-ANCA), among others, are helpful in some patients for differentiating patients with indeterminate colitis and may have some prognostic significance.

The differential diagnosis is broad and includes predominantly infectious causes, ischemia, and long-term NSAID use (**Table 3**).

Treatment is predominantly the purview of the gastroenterologist and primarily involves immunosupressents such as corticosteroids (although these are being used much less commonly), thiopurines, methotrexate, and anti–tumor necrosis factor agents. Other adjunctive agents include 5-aminosalycilates and antibiotics. The goal is foremost to relieve the patient's symptoms and secondarily to induce mucosal healing. If medical therapy fails, surgery often becomes necessary. In UC, total colectomy is curative. Colectomy with ileoanal pouch procedure reduces fertility in women because of pelvic adhesions. Patients with UC who undergo colectomy with a pouch procedure remain at risk for pouchitis; however, this can usually be managed medically. In CD, surgery is used as a last resort, and the least amount of bowel possible is removed to prevent malabsorption.

Summary

IBD, CD and UC, is characterized by inflammation throughout the GI tract. It is often a relapsing, remitting disease. Clinical presentation often includes abdominal pain with bloody diarrhea, although the transmural inflammation in CD can cause fistulizing and stricturing disease. Diagnosis takes into account the clinical picture, serologies, imaging, endoscopic, and pathologic examinations. Treatment revolves around immunosuppressive agents with or without 5-aminosalicylic acids and antibiotics. Surgery can become necessary and is curative in UC but not in CD.

Table 3
Differential diagnosis of IBD

Infectious: Yersinia, Clostridium difficile, tuberculosis	Appendicitis
Diverticulitis	Ischemic colitis
Radiation proctitis	GI malignancies
Irritable bowel syndrome	Endometriosis

Data from Whitehead WE, Drossman DA. Validation of symptom-based diagnostic criteria for irritable bowel syndrome: a critical review. Am J Gastroenterol 2010;105(4):814–20.

Irritable bowel syndrome

Definition: IBS is defined by abdominal pain with altered bowel habits in the absence of an identifiable organic cause.

It is defined by Rome III criteria (**Box 4**).

Pathology is thought to be due to alterations in gut motility, visceral hypersensitivity, intestinal inflammation, and alterations in fecal microflora. Psychosocial dysfunction often exists, although it is not present in all patients. A subset of people have postinfectious IBS, which occurs after acute gastroenteritis and can last for years.

Four types of IBS subtypes exist and are based on stool form.[60]

1. IBS with constipation
2. IBS with diarrhea
3. Mixed IBS
4. Unsubtyped IBS

In patients with typical symptoms and an absence of alarm features, a presumptive diagnosis of IBS can and should be made. IBS is not a diagnosis of exclusion, although disorders that commonly mimic IBS should be considered, such as celiac disease. The presence of alarm features such as advanced age, weight loss, anemia, fever, and rectal bleeding should alert the physician to a possible pathologic cause to the patient's symptoms (although in most cases, an alternative diagnosis is not found). Appropriate laboratory screening tests depend on the predominant bowel pattern and include complete blood count (CBC), basic metabolic panel (BMP), thyroid-stimulating hormone (TSH), celiac serologies, and possibly stool studies. Imaging, such as abdominal radiography, CT-scan, and MRI, rarely adds to the diagnosis. Colonoscopy should be considered in patients with rectal bleeding, advanced age, and family history of colon cancer or to rule out microscopic colitis in the setting of more severe

Box 4
Rome III criteria for diagnosis of IBS

Recurrent abdominal pain or discomfort at least 3 days per month in the last 3 months associated with 2 or more of the following:

1. Improvement with defecation
2. Onset associated with a change in frequency of stool
3. Onset associated with a change in form (appearance of stool)

Data from Talley NJ, American Gastroenterological Association. American Gastroenterological Association medical position statement: evaluation of dyspepsia. Gastroenterology 2005;129(5):1753–5.

watery diarrhea.[60–62] Patients with IBS are actually less likely to have colonic pathology than age-matched controls.

Once a physician has established IBS as a diagnosis, it is important to educate patients on their diagnosis and the likely chronicity of the disease. Reassurance is important, that their disorder is not life threatening and can be successfully treated. Patients should be encouraged to actively participate in the treatment plan. Dietary modifications are helpful with many patients, and specific diets exist if a patient wishes (including a gluten-free diet and the fermentable, oligo-, di-, mono-saccharides and polyols (FODMAPs) diet). Physical activity and stress management have been associated with improved outcomes. Symptomatic treatment of their diarrhea (eg, loperamide) or constipation (eg, polyethylene glycol) remains a cornerstone of initial treatment. Probiotics, including *Bifidobacterium infantis*, improve symptoms in patients with diarrhea or constipation and help bloating. Patients with severe pain, or pain that does not respond to dietary management or anticholinergic medications (eg, dicyclomine or hyoscyamine), should be considered for neuromodulation with low-dose tricyclic antidepressant therapy. Patients with refractory constipation should be considered for pelvic floor dysfunction (dyssynergic defecation). In addition, the chloride channel-2 agonist lubiprostone and the guanylate cyclase C agonist linaclotide improve symptoms in patients with IBS and constipation. The 5HT-3 receptor antagonist alosetron improves the condition of patients with IBS and refractory diarrhea who have failed more conservative therapies.

Complementary therapies such as hypnotherapy and cognitive behavioral therapy have had success rates that are as good as or better than any medication approved for IBS treatment with evidence of long-term efficacy and excellent safety records.

Patients with IBS are more likely to undergo unnecessary surgeries, including cholecystectomy and hysterectomy. Recognizing and treating the symptoms of IBS may avoid these unnecessary surgeries.

Summary

IBS is characterized by pain and alterations in bowel habits in the absence of an identifiable organic cause; it is identified using Rome III criteria. Diagnostic studies center around identifying red flags or worrisome features. Celiac disease should be considered in patients with IBS. Reassurance and education about IBS improve outcomes. Behavioral modifications, symptomatic management, and neuromodulation are the cornerstones of treatment.

REFERENCES

1. Kalloo AN, Kantsevoy S, Kalloo AN, et al. Gallstones and biliary disease. Prim Care 2001;28(3):591. PMID # 11483446.
2. Feldman M, Friedman L. Sleisenger and Fordtran's gastrointestinal and liver disease. Philadelphia: Saunders (Elsevier); 2010.
3. Kiewiet JJ, Leeuwenburgh MM, Bipat S, et al. A systematic review and meta-analysis of diagnostic performance of imaging in acute cholecystitis. Radiology 2012;264(3):708.
4. Papi C, Catarci M, D'Ambrosio L, et al. Timing of cholecytectomy for acute calculouis cholecystitis: a meta-analysis. Am J Gastroenterol 2004;99:147–55.
5. Chandler CF, Lane JS, Ferguson P, et al. Prospective evaluation of early versus delayed laparoscopic cholecystectomy for treatment of acute cholecystitis. Am Surg 2000;66:896–900.

6. Date RS, Kaushal M, Ramesh A. A review of the management of gallstone disease and its complications in pregnancy. Am J Surg 2008;196(4):599.
7. Himal HS. Lindsay ascending cholangitis: surgery versus endoscopic or percutaneous drainage. Surgery 1990;108(4):629–33 [discussion: 633–4].
8. Greenberger N. Current diagnosis and treatment gastroenterology, hepatology, and endoscopy. McGraw Hill, Lange; 2009.
9. Saik RP, Greenburg AG, Farris JM, et al. Spectrum of cholangitis. Am J Surg 1975;130(2):143.
10. Mosler P. Diagnosis and management of acute cholangitis. Curr Gastroenterol Rep 2011;13(2):166–72.
11. Pasanen PA, Partanen KP, Pikkarainen PH, et al. A comparison of ultrasound, computed tomography and endoscopic retrograde cholangiopancreatography in the differential diagnosis of benign and malignant jaundice and cholestasis. Eur J Surg 1993;159(1):23.
12. Becker CD, Grossholz M, Becker M, et al. Choledocholithiasis and bile duct stenosis: diagnostic accuracy of MR cholangiopancreatography. Radiology 1997; 205(2):523.
13. Mahmoud AE, Mendoza A, Meshikhes AN, et al. Clinical spectrum, investigations and treatment of Budd-Chiari syndrome. QJM 1996;89(1):37.
14. DeLeve LD, Valla DC, Garcia-Tsao G. Vascular disorders of the liver, American Association for the Study Liver Diseases Practice Guidelines. Hepatology 2009; 49(5):1729.
15. Fickert P, Ramschak H, Kenner L, et al. Acute Budd-Chiari syndrome with fulminant hepatic failure in a pregnant woman with factor V Leiden mutation. Gastroenterology 1996;111(6):1670.
16. Nelson DB, Yost NP, Cunningham FG. Acute fatty liver of pregnancy: clinical outcomes and expected duration of recovery. Am J Obstet Gynecol 2013; 209(5):456.
17. Wang YR, Richter JE, Dempsey DT. Trends and outcomes of hospitalizations for peptic ulcer disease in the United States, 1993 to 2006. Ann Surg 2010; 251(1):51.
18. Grassi R, Romano S, Pinto A, et al. Gastro-duodenal perforations: conventional plain film, US and CT findings in 166 consecutive patients. Eur J Radiol 2004; 50(1):30.
19. Peery AF, Dellon ES, Lund J, et al. Burden of gastrointestinal disease in the United States: 2012 update. Gastroenterology 2012;143(5):1179–87.e1-3.
20. Forsmark CE, Baillie J, AGA Institute Clinical Practice and Economics Committee, AGA Institute Governing Board. AGA Institute technical review on acute pancreatitis. Gastroenterology 2007;132(5):2022.
21. Swaroop VS, Chari ST, Clain JE. Severe acute pancreatitis. JAMA 2004;291(23): 2865.
22. Banks PA. Acute pancreatitis: diagnosis. In: Lankisch PG, Banks PA, editors. Pancreatitis. New York: Springer-Verlag; 1998. p. 75.
23. Banks PA, Freeman ML. Practice guidelines in acute pancreatitis. Am J Gastroenterol 2006;101(10):2379.
24. Banks PA, Bollen TL, Dervenis C, et al, Acute Pancreatitis Classification Working Group. Classification of acute pancreatitis–2012: revision of the Atlanta classification and definitions by international consensus. Gut 2013;62(1):102.
25. Tenner S, Baillie J, DeWitt J, et al, American College of Gastroenterology. American College of Gastroenterology guideline: management of acute pancreatitis. Am J Gastroenterol 2013;108(9):1400.

26. Addiss DG, Shaffer N, Fowler BS, et al. The epidemiology of appendicitis and appendectomy in the United States. Am J Epidemiol 1990;132(5):910.
27. Wagner JM, McKinney WP, Carpenter JL. Does this patient have appendicitis? JAMA 1996;276(19):1589–94.
28. Anderson RE. Meta-analysis of the clinical and laboratory diagnosis of appendicitis. Br J Surg 2004;91(1):28.
29. Hong JJ, Cohn SM, Ekeh AP, et al, Miami Appendicitis Group. A prospective randomized study of clinical assessment versus computed tomography for the diagnosis of acute appendicitis. Surg Infect (Larchmt) 2003;4(3):231.
30. Mahmoodian S. Appendicitis complicating pregnancy. South Med J 1992;85(1): 19–24.
31. Barkun A, Leontiadis G. Systematic review of the symptom burden, quality of life impairment and costs associated with peptic ulcer disease. Am J Med 2010; 1123(4):358–66.
32. Gururatsakul M, Holloway RH, Talley NJ, et al. Association between clinical manifestations of complicated and uncomplicated peptic ulcer and visceral sensory dysfunction. J Gastroenterol Hepatol 2010;25(6):1162–9.
33. Chey WD, Wong BC. American College of Gastroenterology guideline on the management of *Helicobacter pylori* infection. Am J Gastroenterol 2007;102(8): 1808–25.
34. Dammann HG, Walter TA. Efficacy of continuous therapy for peptic ulcer in controlled clinical trials. Aliment Pharmacol Ther 1993;7(Suppl 2):17–25.
35. Tytgat GN. The Sydney System: endoscopic division. Endoscopic appearances in gastritis/duodenitis. J Gastroenterol Hepatol 1991;6(3):223.
36. Antico A, Tampoia M, Villalta D, et al. Clinical usefulness of the serological gastric biopsy for the diagnosis of chronic autoimmune gastritis. Clin Dev Immunol 2012;2012:520970.
37. Parks TG. Natural history of diverticular disease of the colon. A review of 521 cases. Br Med J 1969;4(5684):639.
38. Nguyen GC, Sam J, Anand N. Epidemiological trends and geographic variation in hospital admissions for diverticulitis in the United States. World J Gastroenterol 2011;17(12):1600–5.
39. Jacobs DO. Clinical practice. Diverticulitis. N Engl J Med 2007;357(20):2057–66.
40. Salzman H, Lillie D. Diverticular disease: diagnosis and treatment. Am Fam Physician 2005;72(7):1229.
41. Regenbogen SE, Hardiman KM, Hendren S, et al. Surgery for diverticulitis in the 21st century: a systematic review. JAMA Surg 2014;149(3):292.
42. McKinsey JF, Gewertz BL. Acute mesenteric ischemia. Surg Clin North Am 1997;77(2):307.
43. American Gastroenterological Association Medical Position Statement. guidelines on intestinal ischemia. Gastroenterology 2000;118(5):951.
44. Kougias P, Lau D, El Sayed HF, et al. Determinants of mortality and treatment outcome following surgical interventions for acute mesenteric ischemia. J Vasc Surg 2007;46(3):467.
45. Acosta S, Alhadad A, Svensson P, et al. Epidemiology, risk and prognostic factors in mesenteric venous thrombosis. Br J Surg 2008;95(10):1245.
46. Miller G, Boman J, Shrier I, et al. Etiology of small bowel obstruction. Am J Surg 2000;180(1):33–6.
47. Markogiannakis H, Messaris E, Dardamanis D, et al. Acute mechanical bowel obstruction: clinical presentation, etiology, management and outcome. World J Gastroenterol 2007;13(3):432.

48. Foster N, McGory ML. Small bowel obstruction: a population-based appraisal. J Am Coll Surg 2006;203(2):170–6.
49. Diehl AK, Sugarek NJ, Todd KH, et al. Clinical evaluation for gallstone disease: of symptoms and signs in diagnosis. Am J Med 1990;89(1):29–33.
50. Lai KC, Lam SK, Chu KM, et al. Lansoprazole reduces ulcer relapse after eradication of *Helicobacter pylori* in nonsteroidal anti-inflammatory drug users–a randomized trial. Aliment Pharmacol Ther 2003;18(8):829–36.
51. Talley NJ, American Gastroentrological Association. American Gastroenterological Association medical position statement: evaluation of dyspepsia. Gastroenterology 2005;129(5):1753.
52. Lacy BE, Talley NJ, Locke GR, et al. Review article: current treatment options and management of functional dyspepsia. Aliment Pharmacol Ther 2012;36:3–15.
53. Steer ML, Waxman I, Freedman S. Chronic pancreatitis. N Engl J Med 1995; 332(22):1482.
54. Layer P, Yamamoto H, Kalthoff L, et al. The different courses of early- and late-onset idiopathic and alcoholic chronic pancreatitis. Gastroenterology 1994;107(5):1481.
55. Etemad B, Whitcomb DC. Chronic pancreatitis: diagnosis, classification, and new genetic developments. Gastroenterology 2001;120(3):682–707.
56. Wallace MB, Hawes RH, Durkalski V, et al. The reliability of EUS for the diagnosis of chronic pancreatitis: interobserver agreement among experienced endosonographers. Gastrointest Endosc 2001;53(3):294–9.
57. Loftus EV Jr. Clinical epidemiology of inflammatory bowel disease: incidence, prevalence, and environmental influences. Gastroenterology 2004;126(6):1504.
58. Podolsky DK. Inflammatory bowel disease. N Engl J Med 2002;347(6):417–29.
59. Silverberg MS, Satsangi J, Ahmad T, et al. Toward an integrated clinical, molecular and serological classification of inflammatory bowel disease: report of a Working Party of the 2005 Montreal World Congress of Gastroenterology. Can J Gastroenterol 2005;19(Suppl A):5A.
60. Zanini B, Ricci C, Bandera F, et al. Incidence of post-infectious irritable bowel syndrome and functional intestinal disorders following a water-borne viral gastroenteritis outbreak. Am J Gastroenterol 2012;107(6):891.
61. O'Connor OJ, McSweeney SE, McWilliams S, et al. Role of radiologic imaging in irritable bowel syndrome: evidence-based review. Radiology 2012;262(2):485.
62. McKenzie YA, Alder A, Anderson W, et al, Gastroenterology Specialist Group of the British Dietetic Association. British Dietetic Association evidence-based guidelines for the dietary management of irritable bowel syndrome in adults. J Hum Nutr Diet 2012;25(3):260–74.

Opioid Use and Depression in Chronic Pelvic Pain

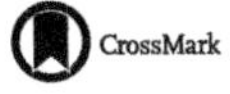

Andrew Steele, MD

KEYWORDS

• Chronic pelvic pain • Addiction • Opioid • Narcotic • Depression

KEY POINTS

- Opioid prescribing is a national epidemic, associated with high rates of diversion of prescription therapeutics.
- Opioid therapy should rarely be initiated for patients with chronic pelvic pain, even in the setting of a referring practice or emergency department.
- Screening tools can help predict and detect opioid addiction and diversion.
- Women on chronic opioid therapy for chronic noncancer pain should be weaned off their medication before attempted conception.
- Women with chronic pain should be screened for depression and treatment or referral provided when positive.

INTRODUCTION

Prescription medication abuse has become a national epidemic. In 2011, more than 238 million narcotic analgesic prescriptions were written, with more attributable deaths than heroin and cocaine combined.[1] According to data from the 2010 National Survey on Drug Use and Health,[2] the nonmedical misuse of prescription psychotherapeutics, including opioids, was the second leading type of illicit drug abuse, behind marijuana. Further data from the Survey found that almost one-third of people aged 12 and over who initiated illicit drug use for the first time began by using a prescription drug nonmedically. In addition, review articles on the use of opioids for chronic pain have found limited data supporting their long-term use in a variety of pain conditions.[3]

Women's health care providers are confronted with several chronic pain syndromes ranging from irritable bowel syndrome, interstitial cystitis and endometriosis, to musculoskeletal pain, vestibulitis, and pelvalgia. Often patients present to the consultant already having received long-term narcotic prescriptions, initiated from other providers. Volkow and McLellan[4] found that the main prescribers of opioids are primary care

The author has nothing to disclose.
Obstetrics, Gynecology and Women's Health, Surgery, Saint Louis University, 6420 Clayton Road, St Louis, MO 63117, USA
E-mail address: steeleac@slu.edu

Obstet Gynecol Clin N Am 41 (2014) 491–501
http://dx.doi.org/10.1016/j.ogc.2014.04.005 **obgyn.theclinics.com**
0889-8545/14/$ – see front matter

providers, followed by dentists and orthopedic surgeons, with the main prescribers for patients aged 10 to 19 being dentists. Emergency room visits also led to significant opioid prescribing. In one large insurance database, it was found that more than 400,000 narcotic prescriptions were written in 2009 through emergency departments for plan enrollees aged 18 to 64. More startling was that 10% of these patients who received narcotic prescriptions did so despite identifiable risk factors for opioid misuse.[5]

Primary care providers have reported unease at chronic opioid prescribing, while simultaneously noting the difficulty of referral to pain management centers.[6] In the author's practice, the patient's access to medication management by trained pain specialists is often limited by insurance considerations as well as the procedural focus (ie, injection therapy) of many pain management physicians.

THE PAIN EXPERIENCE

The experience of pain varies from patient to patient and is a factor of the patient's underlying coping skills, mental health, support, and potential secondary gain.[7] Furthermore, chronic pain and the medications used to treat pain lead to other complications, such as sleeplessness, job performance issues, and relationship issues (**Fig. 1**).

The perception of pain carries 2 components best summed in the legal term, "pain and suffering." The pain component, or sensory-discriminative component, is quantifiable and amenable to therapy. Suffering, or the affective-motivational component, is more difficult to quantify and treat with therapies targeted at the disease process.[7] Thus, one aspect of the physician-patient educational component is that therapy may, "fix your pain but not your suffering." It is important that alternative options for pain control are discussed with the patient. Physicians should be aware of resources in his or her community. Establishing collegial relationships with local counselors, acupuncturists, and pain management specialists allows the obstetrician/gynecologist (OB/GYN) to develop a multidisciplinary approach to the patient with chronic pelvic pain (CPP).

NARCOTIC ACTIONS

Nociceptive (pain) signals are transmitted to the superficial dorsal horn of the brain via sodium-dependent depolarization predominantly via A-δ and C fibers.[8] Opioids have

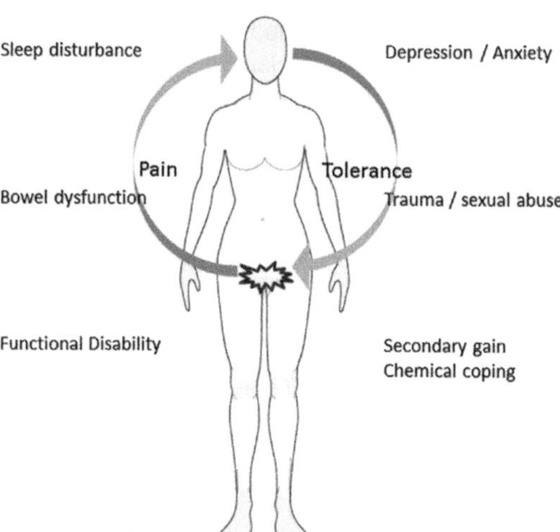

Fig. 1. The interaction of CPP with other psychosocial factors.

their primary effect on mu receptors. These receptors are located in the cortex, thalamus, and periaqueductal gray matter as well as the spinal cord. Two types of mu receptors have been proposed. Mu1 receptors have a high affinity for morphine and its derivatives and are dominant receptors in supraspinal analgesia as well as the development of physical tolerance. Mu2 receptors have a lower affinity to morphine and are implicated in narcotic side effects, such as respiratory depression and constipation.[9] Mu receptors are also involved in the reward response associated with opioid use via increasing dopaminergic release. Medications with the most rapid onset of action tend to cause the most euphoria, and that euphoric reward is the first effect lost with developing tolerance. Thus, patients need increasing doses to achieve the same euphoric reward response. Side effects of opioid medications are generally dose-dependent and include constipation, meiosis, sedation, and respiratory depression.[10]

TOLERANCE, DEPENDENCE, AND ADDICTION

Tolerance, physical dependence, and addiction are not synonymous terms, although all 3 may lead to aberrant medication-taking behaviors (AMTB). Over time, patients on chronic narcotics may develop tolerance to the medication requiring escalating dosages. Patients demonstrating AMTBs because of inadequate analgesia have what is termed pseudo-addiction. Physical dependence represents physiologic adaptation with signs and symptoms of withdrawal if the opioid is abruptly stopped and is an effect of tolerance. Both tolerance and dependence may be anticipated with chronic narcotic use. Addiction manifests with AMTBs representing impaired control over opioid use and a preoccupation with obtaining opioids. In cases of addiction, patients will also continue opioid use despite evidence of harm from the medications, such as, declining function in relationships or work, intoxication, or persistent oversedation.[11] Medication diversion is another concern with narcotic prescribing. Approximately 76% of opioids used for nonmedical purposes were originally prescribed to someone else.[12]

DETECTING “AT-RISK” PATIENTS

Screening tools exist to help determine those patients at higher risk for opioid misuse. A prior history of personal or family history of substance abuse is major risk factor for opioid misuse. Smoking is a significant risk factor for opioid misuse, because up to 95% of patients treated for another substance abuse disorder also smoke.[13] Questionnaires provide a means of assessing for potential opioid misuse. The SOAPP (Screener and Opioid Assessment for Patients with Pain) is a 24-question validated survey in which patients answer questions in domains, such as lifestyle, physician-patient relationship, antisocial behaviors, medication-use behaviors, psychiatric disorders, and psychosocial difficulties.[14,15] An abbreviated, 14-question version has also been reported.[13] Another potentially useful questionnaire is the Opioid Risk Tool (ORT). Both elevated as well as low scores on the ORT have been associated with a high and low likelihood of demonstrating later AMTBs, respectively.[16] Although questionnaires are safe and easy to administer, a recent review has shown variable utility in the identification of at-risk patients, with studies showing a mixed picture with overall weak associations between positive screens and future medication misuse.[17]

AMTB

Aberrant drug-related behaviors can be markers of prescription medication abuse or diversion (**Fig. 2**). These behaviors may include patients receiving narcotics from

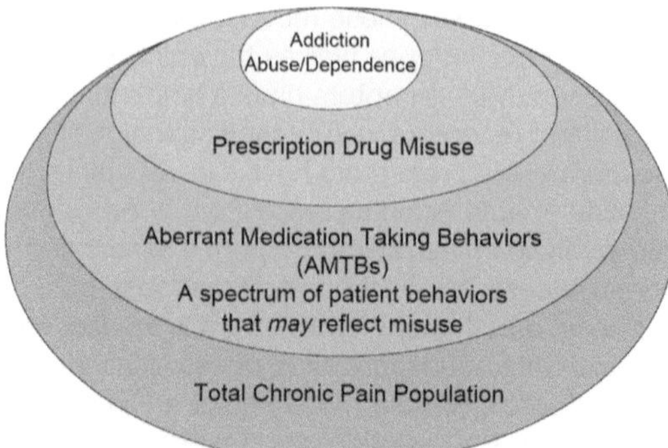

Fig. 2. The spectrum of opioid tolerance and abuse disorders. (*From* Alford D. Chronic pain and opioid risk management. Chief Resident Immersion Training (CRIT) Program in Addiction Medicine, Boston University. 2010. Available at: http://www.bumc.bu.edu/care/files/2010/09/11.-ALFORD-Chronic-Pain-and-Opioid-Risk-Management.pdf. Accessed February 15, 2014; with permission.)

multiple providers simultaneously; requesting specific, short-acting medications; or relating allergies to nonnarcotic pain medications. These behaviors often serve as "yellow flags" or "red flags" to the clinician.[18] It is important to remember that all patients with AMTBs are not addicted to opioids, nor even misusing them. Rather, there is a spectrum of use in which concern needs to be raised when AMBTs are demonstrated (**Box 1**).

Studies have found significant gender differences in AMBTs. Simoni-Wastila and colleagues[19,20] have noted that women have significantly higher rates of nonmedical use of prescription opioids compared with men, noting that women are 48% more likely than men to use any abusable prescription drug, when controlled for demographics, health and economic status, and diagnosis.[20] Women are also more likely to supplement their nonmedical use with other prescription drugs, such as anxiolytics or sedatives.[21,22]

However, aberrant and drug-seeking behaviors have another, more subtle effect. The patient who calls frequently for refills, or calls after hours or on weekends, also places tremendous strain on a doctor's office personnel, staff, or colleagues. This

Box 1
Aberrant drug-seeking behaviors

Warning signs of addiction

- Multiple lost or stolen prescriptions
- Failure to comply with monitoring (random drug screens)
- Current use of alcohol or illicit drugs
- Multiple prescriptions from different physicians or pharmacies
- Forging, selling, or stealing prescriptions

Possible misuse, logistically burdensome

- Calls after hours/weekends for refills
- Requesting narcotic adjustment or changes by phone
- Narcotic hoarding/overutilization

practice, in turn, harms the physician-patient relationship and may ultimately lead to severing of care in a patient who legitimately needs assistance. Strategies to minimize AMTBs and limit adverse narcotic events will benefit both the patient and the provider.

OPIOID MANAGEMENT STRATEGIES

There is scant evidence supporting the role of opioid therapy in chronic pain, and risks to the patient from narcotics are not insignificant.[23] As such, providers should be hesitant to initiate any narcotic therapy for CPP, even in the initial evaluation phase while tests are pending. In patients presenting with CPP, simple screening questions may help identify patients at risk for opioid misuse.

Several strategies exist to help minimize AMBTs and decrease the likelihood of abuse or redirection (**Boxes 2** and **3**). Patient contracts are widely used for patients seeking long-term opioid prescriptions. Often, patients will require a separate visit to undergo screening and to review and initiate the contract; remember that the opioid need itself can represent a disease state that needs the same attention as the gynecologic condition. Contracts spell out policies and expectations but must be used in conjunction with a clear overall strategy for narcotic use. Simply listing the AMBTs that will cause the patient to be disengaged from the practice is inadequate. Instead, expectations for periodic reassessment of the efficacy of the pain management, practice policies regarding refills, and exit strategies for discontinuing these medications should be spelled out at initiation of the therapy. Some suggestions are listed in **Box 2**.

PERIODIC REASSESSMENT

Periodic reassessment in the office is a valuable method for ensuring adequate analgesia and limiting abuse. Several tools are available for clinical use.

Pill Counts

Pill counts aid in assessing overuse, underuse as well as diversion. Pill counts may be especially useful for the patient who calls before the scheduled renewal complaining of intolerance or ineffectiveness of a current medication and requesting a prescription change. In general, these patients are asked to schedule a visit to discuss the need for medication adjustment, to assess for new conditions that would lead to a deterioration in their pain control, and to undergo pill counting of the unused medication. In patients being managed on fentanyl patches, the used patches should be returned because a small amount of fentanyl could be still be extracted.

Box 2
PEG physician-administered pain score

1. What number best describes your pain on average in the past week? (0 No pain to 10 pain as bad as you can imagine)
2. What number best describes how, during the past week, pain has interfered with your enjoyment of life? (0 Does not interfere to 10 completely interferes)
3. What number best describes how, during the past week, pain has interfered with your general activity? (0 Does not interfere to 10 completely interferes)

Adapted from Krebs EE, Lorenz KA, Bair MJ, et al. Development and initial validation of the PEG, a three-item scale assessing pain intensity and interference. J Gen Intern Med 2009;24(6):733–8.

Box 3
Strategies to prevent abuse and redirection of prescribed opioids

Strategies to prevent abuse and redirection
- Patient contracts
- Single provider and pharmacy for all opioid prescriptions
- Urine drug testing
- Regular validated questionnaires
- Pill counts

Strategies to prevent abuse and minimize practice impact
- Concurrent use of complementary and alternative therapies
  - Acupuncture
  - NSAIDs
  - Stress management
  - Counseling
- Regularly scheduled follow-up visits specifically addressing pain management
- Communication of office practice expectations
  - No after-hours refill requests
  - No medication dose/frequency adjustment by phone
  - No phone replacement of lost/stolen prescriptions

Urine Drug Testing

Urine drug testing may be accomplished in an office-based practice.[24] Urine drug testing may sometimes detect unrecognized abuse or misuse even in "model" patients. Katz and Fanciullo[25] reported findings that 21% of chronic pain patients had positive urine drug screens despite demonstrating no ABMTs. A negative urine drug screen in a patient on chronic opioid therapy may represent unintentional underutilization, diversion, or disingenuous specimen substitution. Although commonly recommended in discussions of opioid prescribing, the practice raises many questions. Medical urine drug testing is not a forensic process. At the same time, the practitioner must use judgment in evaluating results. For instance, will the specimen collection be supervised? Will temperature or creatinine be checked to discourage substitution? What are the limitations, such as cross-reactivity, of the specific urine drug test and laboratory you will be using?[26]

Patient Questionnaires

As with other decisions in medicine, the ongoing benefits of chronic opioid therapy should be weighed against the risks of its use. The "4 A's" of the therapy should be periodically assessed and include evaluating *A*nalgesia, *A*ctivities of daily living, *A*dverse events, and *A*berrant drug-taking behaviors.[27] One way to assess the ongoing utility of the therapy, as well as the development of tolerance or addiction, is with questionnaires. These questionnaires can be either patient-administered or physician-administered. The Current Opioid Misuse Measure is a patient self-administered, validated questionnaire. The 17-point list has a negative sensitivity of 77% but a specificity of only 66%, suggesting that not all screen positives will be misusing medications.[28] Another physician-administered questionnaire is the PEG (pain, enjoyment, general activity) Scale.[29] Patients rate the following on a 0 to 10 scale with 10 being most severe or disruptive (see **Box 2**).

It should be noted that these questionnaires differ from previously mentioned screening strategies for detecting possible abuse; instead, they represent methods of assessing the effectiveness and negative impact of the ongoing opioid treatment.

EXIT STRATEGIES

Exit strategies should be addressed early in the relationship as part of the informed consent process. The patient should be made aware of the possibility that medication therapy will be discontinued or modulated if the risks of medication use to the patient outweigh the benefits. This discussion should be kept separate from threats to disengage the patient from care. Even when exiting from opioid prescribing, the OB/GYN should focus on ongoing treatments for the disease process or processes.[18] Referral should be considered for more specialized care at tertiary referral centers as well as for addiction evaluation and treatment if needed.

OPIOIDS AND PREGNANCY

One special population confronting the obstetrician is the pregnant patient presenting on chronic opioid therapy. Although some concern existed in animal studies, until recently standard texts in the field reported no definite association between the development of congenital anomalies in women with the use of morphine derivatives, including codeine, oxycodone, or hydromorphone.[30] More recent large studies, however, have called the safety of opioids in pregnancy into question. Broussard and colleagues,[31] using the Birth Defects Prevention Database, found statistically significant increases in the following anomalies in mothers using opioids in the peri-conceptual period (1-month preconception) and first trimester. These anomalies included conoventricular septal defects (odds ratio [OR], 2.7; 95% confidence interval [CI], 1.1–6.3), atrioventricular septal defects (OR, 2.0; 95% CI, 1.2–3.6), hypoplastic left heart syndrome (OR, 2.4; 95% CI, 1.4–4.1), spina bifida (OR, 2.0; 95% CI, 1.3–3.2), and gastroschisis (OR, 1.8; 95% CI, 1.1–2.9).[31] The Swedish Medical Register presented data on more than 7000 infants born to mothers who reported the use of opioids during early pregnancy. In that study, the only anomaly reaching statistical significance was pes equinovarus in women taking tramadol.[32] Studies using databases on the effects of opioid medications during pregnancy are often confounded by polysubstance use in subjects, as well as the retrospective nature of the data collection. Nonetheless, women requiring chronic opioid therapy should be encouraged to wean off their medication before attempted conception. In those women who present already on chronic narcotic therapy, referral to maternal fetal medicine and pain management specialists may be indicated.

ABUSE, DEPRESSION, AND CHRONIC PAIN

The relationship between women suffering from CPP and prior traumatic events has been well established.[33–35] Up to 50% of women with CPP in a referral population had a history of prior sexual or physical abuse. In that series, Meltzer-Brody and colleagues[36] found that 1 in 3 women also demonstrated evidence of posttraumatic stress disorder. The association between domestic physical and sexual abuse in dysfunctional households may make the contribution of either component difficult to determine[33,37,38]; however, women with CPP have been clearly found to have a higher incidence of early (under age 15) sexual abuse as well as severe childhood sexual abuse.[33,39]

Depression is much more common in women with CPP. Walker and colleagues[35] found that women with CPP had a higher incidence of several psychiatric conditions, including major depression, substance abuse, adult sexual dysfunction, and somatization.[35] This higher incidence of psychiatric conditions was the case despite similar degrees of intra-abdominal pathologic abnormality. The underlying associations between chronic pain and depression are complex. The 2 conditions may coexist because underlying adverse life experiences predispose women to both conditions. Depression may occur because the underlying pain condition leads to vegetative changes in function manifesting as depression. Finally, the strong association may exist because women with depression have a greater sensitization to noxious stimuli and diminished neuroendocrine coping mechanisms. In most cases, it may be difficult to tell which condition predisposed a given patient to the other.[40] Research has suggested that the loss of norepinephrine and serotonin in the periaqueductal gray matter can occur with ongoing painful stimuli. This area of the brain is thought to be responsible for the modulation of pain, so that loss of modulatory function here leads to an increase in attention to and emotional association with pain.[41] Thus, from the standpoint of neuropathology, there may not be a distinction that can be made between cause and consequence.

Women presenting with CPP should be specifically questioned about a past history of sexual abuse or trauma, especially in childhood. Screening for posttraumatic stress disorder should also be undertaken.[36] Several simple screening tools exist for the clinician's use. The main key is that this is done early in the therapeutic relationship. Waiting to delve into these issues until the patient has undergone a series of negative tests may send a message to the patient that the psychosocial issues are secondary or untreatable. Screening questions may be introduced by discussing the holistic understanding of the patient to include medical, spiritual, and mental facets.

There is limited evidence to support the use of antidepressants in women specifically for CPP.[42] In women with CPP and associated depression, treatment of their depression may be initiated during the evaluation of their pain. Tricyclic antidepressants, such as amitriptyline or nortriptyline, and serotonin-norepinephrine reuptake inhibitors, such as duloxetine, are commonly used antidepressants in patients with other chronic, non-pelvic pain syndromes.[43] When initiating antidepressants, the clinician should "start low and go slow."[43] Care should be taken to evaluate for suicidal ideation. A review of potential medication interactions should be completed based on the specific medication prescribed. Clinicians unfamiliar with treating depression should consider referral. In addition, nonmedical therapy, including psychologic evaluation and counseling, should be offered.

SUMMARY

OB/GYN physicians frequently deal with chronic pain patients. Whenever possible, initiating narcotics in patients with CPP should be avoided, even when the physician is covering a patient with chronic pain in the emergency department. When patients present already on narcotics, the patient may have already been formally or informally disengaged from the referring practice, leaving the OB/GYN in the unenviable position of needing to deal with the condition as well as the opioid requirements that other physicians have established. When the OB/GYN becomes the primary prescriber, establishing boundaries and goals is important. In those cases, screening for addiction risks and completing a pain contract should be considered, along with developing a plan for periodic reassessments.

REFERENCES

1. Manchikanti L, Helm S 2nd, Fellows B, et al. Opioid epidemic in the United States. Pain Physician 2012;15(Suppl 3):ES9–38.
2. Substance Abuse and Mental Health Services Administration. Results from the 2010 National Survey on Drug Use and Health: Summary of National Findings. NSDUH Series H-41, HHS Publication No. (SMA) 11-4658. Rockville (MD): Substance Abuse and Mental Health Services Administration; 2011. Available at: www.samhsa.gov/data/NSDUH/2k10NSDUH/2k10Results.pdf.
3. Von Korff M, Kolodny A, Deyo RA, et al. Long-term opioid therapy reconsidered. Ann Intern Med 2011;155(5):325–8.
4. Volkow ND, McLellan TA. Curtailing diversion and abuse of opioid analgesics without jeopardizing pain treatment. JAMA 2011;305(13):1346–7.
5. Logan J, Liu Y, Paulozzi L, et al. Opioid prescribing in emergency departments: the prevalence of potentially inappropriate prescribing and misuse. Med Care 2013;51(8):646–53.
6. Barry DT, Irwin KS, Jones ES, et al. Opioids, chronic pain, and addiction in primary care. J Pain 2010;11(12):1442–50.
7. Savage SR, Kirsh KL, Passik SD. Challenges in using opioids to treat pain in persons with substance use disorders. Addict Sci Clin Pract 2008;4(2):4–25.
8. Giordano J. The neurobiology of nociceptive and anti-nociceptive systems. Pain Physician 2005;8(3):277–90.
9. Koneru A, Satyanarayana S, Rizwan S. Endogenous opioids: their physiological role and receptors. Global Journal Pharmacology 2009;3(3):149–53.
10. Yaksh T, Wallace MS. Opioids, analgesia, and pain management. In: Brunton LL, Chabner BA, Knollmann BC, editors. Goodman & Gilman's the pharmacological basis of therapeutics. 12th edition. New York: McGraw-Hill Medical. Available at: http://accessmedicine.mhmedical.com/content.aspx?bookid=374&Sectionid=41266224. Accessed May 30, 2014.
11. Miller SC, Frankowski D. Prescription opioid use disorder: a complex clinical challenge. Current Psychiatry 2012;11(8):15–22. Available at: http://www.currentpsychiatry.com/index.php?id=22661&tx_ttnews(tt_news)=176994.
12. U.S. Department of Health and Human Services. Substance Abuse and Mental Health Services Administration. Office of Applied Studies. Results from the 2009 national survey on drug use and health: volume I. Available at: http://www.samhsa.gov/data/NSDUH/2k9NSDUH/2k9Results.htm. Accessed June 20, 2012.
13. Akbik H, Butler SF, Budman SH, et al. Validation and clinical application of the Screener and Opioid Assessment for Patients with Pain (SOAPP). J Pain Symptom Manage 2006;32(3):287–93.
14. Butler SF, Fernandez K, Benoit C, et al. Validation of the Revised Screener and Opioid Assessment for Patients with Pain (SOAPP-R). J Pain 2008;9(4):360–72.
15. Butler SF, Budman SH, Fernandez K, et al. Screener and opioid assessment measure for patients with chronic pain. Pain 2004;112(1–2):65–75.
16. Webster LR, Webster RM. Predicting aberrant behaviors in opioid treated patients: preliminary validation of the Opioid Risk Tool. Pain Med 2005;6(6):432–42.
17. Chou R, Fanciullo GJ, Fine PG, et al. Opioids for chronic noncancer pain: prediction and identification of aberrant drug-related behaviors: a review of the evidence for an American Pain Society and American Academy of Pain Medicine clinical practice guideline. Pain 2009;10(2):131–46.
18. Alford D. Chronic pain and opioid risk management. Chief Resident Immersion Training (CRIT) Program in Addiction Medicine, Boston University 2010. Available

at: http://www.bumc.bu.edu/care/files/2010/09/11.-ALFORD-Chronic-Pain-and-Opioid-Risk-Management.pdf. Accessed February 15, 2014.

19. Simoni-Wastila L, Ritter G, Strickler G. Gender and other factors associated with the nonmedical use of abusable prescription drugs. Subst Use Misuse 2004; 39(1):1–23.
20. Simoni-Wastila L. The use of abusable prescription drugs: the role of gender. J Womens Health Gend Based Med 2000;9(3):289–97.
21. Back SE, Payne RA, Waldrop AE, et al. Prescription opioid aberrant behaviors: a pilot study of gender differences. Clin J Pain 2009;25(6):477–84.
22. Tetrault JM, Desai RA, Becker WC, et al. Gender and non-medical use of prescription opioids: results from a national US survey. Addiction 2008;103(2): 258–68.
23. Manchikanti L, Abdi S, Atluri S, et al. American Society of Interventional Pain Physicians (ASIPP) Guidelines for responsible opioid prescribing in chronic non-cancer pain: Part I – Evidence assessment. Pain Physician 2012;15(Suppl 3):S1–65.
24. Christo PJ, Manchikanti L, Ruan X, et al. Urine drug testing in chronic pain. Pain Physician 2011;14(2):123–43.
25. Katz N, Fanciullo GJ. Role of urine toxicology testing in the management of chronic opioid therapy. Clin J Pain 2002;18(Suppl 4):S76–82.
26. Starrels JL, Becker WC, Alford DP, et al. Systematic review: treatment agreements and urine drug testing to reduce opioid misuse in patients with chronic pain. Ann Intern Med 2010;152(11):712–20.
27. Passik SD. Issues in long-term opioid therapy: unmet needs, risks, and solutions. Mayo Clin Proc 2009;84(7):593–601.
28. Current Opioid Misuse Measure. Available at: http://nationalpaincentre.mcmaster.ca/documents/comm_sample_watermarked.pdf. Accessed February 15, 2014.
29. Krebs EE, Lorenz KA, Bair MJ, et al. Development and initial validation of the PEG, a three-item scale assessing pain intensity and interference. J Gen Intern Med 2009;24(6):733–8.
30. Reuvers M, Schaefer C. Analgesics and anti-inflammatory drugs. In: Briggs, Freeman, Yaffe, editors. Drugs during pregnancy and lactation. 9th edition. Amsterdam: Elsevier; 2007. p. 33–7 Ebook.
31. Broussard CS, Rasmussen SA, Reefhuis J, et al. National Birth Defects Prevention Study. Maternal treatment with opioid analgesics and risk for birth defects. Am J Obstet Gynecol 2011;204(4):314.e1–11.
32. Kallen B, Borg N, Reis M. The use of central nervous system active drugs during pregnancy. Pharmaceuticals 2013;6:1221–86.
33. Lampe A, Solder E, Ennemoser A, et al. Chronic pelvic pain and previous sexual abuse. Obstet Gynecol 2000;96:929–33.
34. Golding JM, Wilsnack SC, Learman LA. Prevalence of sexual assault history among women with common gynecologic symptoms. Am J Obstet Gynecol 1998;179:1013–9.
35. Walker EA, Katon W, Harrop-Griffiths J, et al. Relationship of chronic pelvic pain to psychiatric diagnoses and childhood sexual abuse. Am J Psychiatry 1988;145: 75–80.
36. Meltzer-Brody S, Leserman J, Zolnoun D, et al. Trauma and posttraumatic stress disorder in women with chronic pelvic pain. Obstet Gynecol 2007; 4(109):902–8.
37. Rapkin AJ, Kames LD, Darke LL, et al. History of physical and sexual abuse in women with chronic pelvic pain. Obstet Gynecol 1990;76(1):92–6.

38. Drossman DA, Leserman J, Nachman G, et al. Sexual and physical abuse in women with functional or organic gastrointestinal disorders. Ann Intern Med 1990;113(11):828–33.
39. Walker EA, Katon WJ, Hansom J, et al. Medical and psychiatric symptoms in women with childhood sexual abuse. Psychosom Med 1992;54(6):658–64.
40. Ghally A, Chien P. Chronic pelvic pain: clinical dilemma or clinician's nightmare. Sex Transm Infect 2000;76:419–25.
41. Bair MJ, Robinson RL, Eckert GJ, et al. Impact of pain on depression treatment response in primary care. Psychosom Med 2004;66:17–22.
42. Cheong YC, Smotra G, Williams AC. Non-surgical interventions for the management of chronic pelvic pain. Cochrane Database Syst Rev 2014;(3):CD008797.
43. Schultz E, Malone DA. A practical approach to prescribing antidepressants. Cleve Clin J Med 2013;80(10):625–31.

Complementary and Alternative Medications for Chronic Pelvic Pain

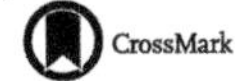

Fah Che Leong, MS, MD

KEYWORDS

- Complementary medicine • Alternative medicine • Chronic pelvic pain
- Interstitial cystitis • Endometriosis

KEY POINTS

- The use of complementary and alternative medicine is common and can account for as much as 11.2% of out-of-pocket expenditures for medical care.
- Patients seek information from peers as well as physicians with regard to alternative medical treatments.
- Rigorous controlled studies of the use of alternative medicine for pelvic pain are lacking.
- Some complementary medicine adjuncts such as dietary supplementation show some promise, but more studies are necessary.

INTRODUCTION

Chronic pelvic pain is a common condition that has significant clinical as well as economic impact. Medical and surgical management may be inadequate in either improving or eliminating the patient's pain, and many patients as well as practitioners have considered the use of complementary and alternative treatments. The causes for chronic pelvic pain can be structural or functional, and frequently can be both. There can be significant difficulty in finding the causes affecting the individual, and, when sufficiently frustrated, patients and physicians turn to alternatives. In 2007, 38.1 million adults made 354 million visits to alternative medicine practitioners and spent $34 billion for all medical conditions.[1] According to the US National Center for Complementary and Alternative Medicine (NCCAM) of the National Institutes of Health, complementary medicine costs are about 11.2% of the total out-of-pocket expenditures on health care. Chronic pelvic pain can affect 14.7% of women between the ages of 18 and 50 years, with an estimated direct cost of $881.5 million.[2] In an earlier study,

Obstetrics Gynecology and Women's Health, Saint Louis University, 6420 Clayton Road, St Louis, MO 63117, USA
E-mail address: leongfc@slu.edu

Obstet Gynecol Clin N Am 41 (2014) 503–510
http://dx.doi.org/10.1016/j.ogc.2014.05.001 **obgyn.theclinics.com**
0889-8545/14/$ – see front matter

12% of all hysterectomies and up to 40% of all laparoscopies were performed for chronic pelvic pain in women.[3] Although the focus of this article is pelvic pain in women, it can be difficult to differentiate pelvic pain from pain in other areas in the low back and low abdomen. Other common conditions include low back pain, arthritic pain, neuropathic pain, and conditions such as fibromyalgia, irritable bowel disease, chronic fatigue syndrome, vulvodynia, and rectal pain. Any patient may have more than one coexisting chronic pain condition. It is as difficult for the practitioner to tease out the nuances of the patient's complaints as it is for the patient to avoid self-diagnosis. At the time of writing, there were more than 5 million hits on a Google search for chronic pelvic pain, more than 4 million for treatment of chronic pelvic pain, and 1.4 million for alternative treatments for chronic pelvic pain. There were 234,000 hits from a search for a forum to discuss pelvic pain with other patients (https://www.google.com/#q=forum+pelvic+pain).

Complementary and alternative medicine (CAM) options that are most commonly sought are dietary supplements and herbs, acupuncture, mind/body medicine, and mind/body manipulative methods.

MANAGEMENT GOALS

The difficulty in treating patients with chronic pelvic pain is exacerbated by differences in expectations. Patients expect a cure, and cures are rare. Patients seek care with new providers out of frustration because of a lack of improvement or perceived degree of improvement. It is important to set realistic expectations for the treatment. Even with accurate diagnosis and effective treatment, cure (to the degree of never having the pain again) is rare.[4] Specific goals must be discussed, and this may be difficult if treatment involves more than one discipline. It is important for the treatment team to communicate with each other and with the patient. It is also important for the team to concentrate on the complementary portion of CAM instead of the alternative portion.

HERBAL AND DIETARY STRATEGIES

Dietary Changes

Up to 90% of patients with interstitial cystitis report sensitivities to foods and drink. Common irritants include coffee, tea, citrus, tomatoes, alcohol, and vitamin C. Patients can benefit from finding their own sensitivities and the use of a symptom diary is helpful. Patients are asked to diary their symptoms, menstrual cycle if indicated, emotional state, foods, and drinks over a month. They can also be provided with a list of possible dietary irritants, and be instructed on an elimination diet in which they ingest none of the possible irritants, adding them in stepwise to see the effect of the addition.[5] Although it is logical to presume that dietary changes affect urinary pain, they have also been studied in other areas of pelvic pain. Improvement of pain was reported by 75% of patients who were placed on a gluten-free diet and followed for 12 months.[6] In patients with endometriosis, the use of the antioxidant vitamins E and C improved the pain in 43% of patients, with a concomitant finding of a decrease in peritoneal fluid inflammatory markers.[7]

Phytotherapy (Herbal Medicine)

NCCAM began funding clinical trials in herbal medicine in 2002. Herbal medicine is widely used all over the world, and, in 2007, of the 40% of adults who used CAM, 17.7% used so-called natural products or herbal medications.[8]

Of the $34 billion spent on CAM, $14.8 billion was spent on natural products.[1]

Calcium Glycerophosphate

Seventy-five percent of patients surveyed rated the use of calcium glycerophosphate (Prelief; AKPharma) as helpful in patients with interstitial cystitis.[9] In an earlier study, patients were instructed to use it before meals for 4 weeks. A decrease in severity was noted in more than 40% of the respondents when used with pizza, coffee, acidic fruit, spicy foods, and tomato-based foods, and up to 30% with carbonated drinks, alcohol, and chocolate.[10]

CystoProtek (Meda Consumer Healthcare)

This is an oral supplement containing glucosamine, chondroitin, hyaluronate, quercetin, olive kernel extract, and rutin. In an uncontrolled study, 252 patients who had failed other treatments were studied for up to 12 months. The women experienced a 49% improvement, measured via a visual analog scale.[11]

Intravesical Instillations Not Approved by the US Food and Drug Administration

Many physicians already use combinations of varying contents including heparin, steroid, sodium bicarbonate, and local anesthetic as rescue instillations. There are several products available in Europe that are used for this purpose (dimethyl sulfoxide is the only product approved by the US Food and Drug Administration for this indication in the United States). Hyaluronic acid, available as an instillation agent with the brand name Cystistat (Mylan Pharma), when used in a small number of patients, showed decreases in nocturia (40%) and pain (30%).[12] Other studies have found similar results but used small numbers of patients.[13,14] However, in forum postings, patients have been advised by their peers to obtain these medications from Canada. Other such commercially branded instillations available in foreign markets include Gepan (Pohl-Boskamp; chondroitin sulfate 0.2%), Uracyst (Tribute Pharmaceuticals; chondroitin sulfate 2%), iAluril (Institut Biochemique SA; hyaluronic acid 1.6% and chondroitin sulfate 2%), Hyacyst (Syner-Med; hyaluronic acid solution), and Cystilieve (Medicines By Design Ltd; lidocaine and sodium bicarbonate).

Quercetin

Quercetin is a bioflavonoid found in red wine, green tea, and onions. It reduces inflammation via the inhibition of the production of cytokines interleukin (IL)-6, IL-8, and tumor necrosis factor. Many of the studies using quercetin are of men with pelvic pain attributed to chronic prostatitis.[15] A form of quercetin is available as Cysta-Q (Farr Labs) and has been used for interstitial cystitis. In an open-label study, 22 patients were given 1 capsule twice a day for 4 weeks. In these patients, pain and symptom indices improved.[16]

Marshmallow Root

Although there are no rigorous studies on the use of marshmallow root for pelvic pain, advice on its use is commonly found in Internet forums. It is thought to reduce pain and inflammation, and has been used for more than 2000 years.

Dextroamphetamine Sulfate

All the literature for the use of amphetamines for pelvic pain and interstitial cystitis come from the laboratory of Dr Jerome Check. All 9 citations listed are case reports but the premise that defects in the sympathetic nervous system contributes to pelvic pain is intriguing.[17–19] Complex regional pain syndrome has been thought to be sympathetically mediated,[20] and similarly patients with chronic pelvic pain without discernible anatomic problems are often thought to have neuropathic pain. However, controlled studies are lacking.

Pollen Extract

Pollen extract has been used for chronic pelvic pain for more than 40 years, but most of the literature has been in men. It is available as a dietary supplement under a variety of trade names, such as Cernilton, Prostat/Poltit, and Pollstimol. The main components, cernitin T60 and cernitin GBX have shown spasmolytic and antiinflammatory properties in animal and in-vitro studies. In a recent small study, 90% of the participants reported less pain and increased quality of life.[21] In a controlled study, 73% of the treatment arm showed improvement, compared with 36% in the control arm.[22]

Cannabinoids

Cannabinoid CB-1 receptors are found in the mouse urinary bladder and, as they are activated, bladder activity is modulated.[23] In a study in which bladder biopsies were taken from patients with painful bladder syndrome (PBS) and idiopathic detrusor overactivity (IDO), there was a significant increase of CB-1-immunoreactive suburothelial nerve fibers in PBS and IDO. Patients with chronic pain who were already on narcotics and were given vaporized cannabis showed an average of 27% decrease in pain without any increase in narcotic use.[24]

NONPHARMACOLOGIC STRATEGIES

Acupuncture

Acupuncture is among the oldest healing practices in the world. Thin needles are used to stimulate specific points in the body. The traditional Chinese medicine theory states that this regulates the flow of qi or vital energy that flows along meridians in the body. The most common use for acupuncture is for pain, with back pain being the most common indication. There is difficulty in creating studies with controls for acupuncture, and there may be a significant placebo effect in patients. In a study of men with chronic pelvic pain, acupuncture was controlled using sham acupuncture (needles placed 1 cm away from the acupuncture point). Seventy-three percent of the patients having acupuncture showed improvement, compared with 47% with sham acupuncture.[25] In an analysis of studies of acupuncture for endometriosis, only 1 of 24 studies met the investigators' criteria for a controlled study with adequate diagnostic studies and outcome measures. Auricular acupuncture reduced dysmenorrhea in 92% of patients.[26] Perhaps just as important is the patients' attitude toward the treatment. In a 2007 study, participants who expected acupuncture to relieve pain experienced significantly more pain relief.[27]

Hypnosis

Hypnosis has been used in a variety of pain conditions but studies for specific conditions are few. It has been studied for cancer pain, headaches, low back pain, fibromyalgia, sickle cell disease, and even temporomandibular joint syndrome. Some of the difficulty with extrapolating the results is lack of standardization for hypnosis, small studies, and variables including instructions for self-hypnosis. Many studies use imagery and relaxation techniques. There are some promising data, but better studies are needed.[28] In a study of men with chronic pelvic pain, 16 men were taught self-hypnosis. After 1 month, 47% reported moderate to marked improvement of symptoms, and, after 6 months, 36% continued to have that improvement. However, the investigators stated that the selected participants had moderate to high hypnotic ability, as identified with the Tellegen Absorption Scale, so those with low hypnotic ability were excluded.[29] The sessions were highly individualized so it is difficult to generalize the study to other populations.

Hyperbaric Oxygen

The premise for using hyperbaric oxygen therapy is that interstitial cystitis is perhaps caused by a relative ischemia leading to lower bladder vascular perfusion and pain. With this in mind, the investigators embarked on a pilot study of 6 patients. The treatment was well tolerated, and 4 of 6 patients rated themselves as improved.[30] The investigators then did a sham-controlled, double-blinded study with 21 total patients with only 3 of the 14 patients in the treatment arm improving.[31] An uncontrolled study from Japan showed improvement in 7 of 11 patients who were refractory to other treatments.[32]

Extracorporeal Shock Wave Lithotripsy

Extracorporeal shock wave lithotripsy (ESWL) was found incidentally to improve chronic pelvic pain in men during treatment of urolithiasis. The mechanism is unknown. In a randomized sham-controlled study, 60 patients were divided and treated once weekly for a month, and followed for 12 weeks after treatment was started. ESWL was administered to the perineum without anesthesia. All the patients in the treated arm showed a significant improvement in pain, quality of life, and voiding. There were no side effects noted.[33] In another randomized sham-controlled study with 40 patients, improvement in quality of life and chronic prostatitis symptom index scores were noted.[34] Whether these results are applicable to women is unknown.

Meditation

The most common mind-body therapy is meditation. Most patients use mind-body therapy in combination with traditional medicine and often in consultation with their physician (80% of patients had discussed this with their physician).[35] The philosophy of meditation has its roots in Buddhism. The 2 most common forms of meditation used in clinical relaxation are transcendental meditation (TM) and mindfulness. TM involves concentrating on a mantra (a repetition of a sound, word, or phrase), and mindfulness involves being aware of one's thoughts and letting go of those without emotional attachments.[36] A cross-sectional study of 13 highly trained Zen meditators showed that they had low sensitive to pain, and experienced analgesic effects during Zen meditation.[37] In a pilot study of women with chronic pelvic pain, the women who completed the study had significant improvement in pain scores, physical function, and mental health. However, only 12 of 22 enrolled subjects completed the study.

SUMMARY

Part of the allure of CAM is that many of them do not require prescription by a physician. Another part is the patient's dissatisfaction with current treatment. Even in the best of circumstances, patients with chronic pelvic pain are not cured, but are in good control. Some of what they choose are recommendations by peers, some from their physicians, and some from overpromises in advertisements. In a survey of the use of complementary medicine for interstitial cystitis, one of the most frequent recommenders (55%) were physicians or their office staff.[9] However, this study includes recommendations for dietary changes (avoidance of dietary irritants) and physical therapy, which are more mainstream and also found in American Urological Association guidelines. Research is limited, and studies with good results often are case studies or small uncontrolled series. In a survey of patients by the Interstitial Cystitis Association, the only alternative treatment rated helpful by a significant number of patients was calcium glycerophosphate (Prelief).[9] The therapies discussed are adjuncts and complementary rather than the primary treatments used by patients. Some of the current publications suggest that they may be helpful, but carefully controlled studies are needed.

REFERENCES

1. Nahin RL, Barnes PM, Stussman BJ, et al. Costs of complementary and alternative medicine (CAM) and frequency of visits to CAM practitioners. Hyattsville (MD): US Department of Health and Human Services, Centers for Disease Control and Prevention, National Center for Health Statistics, 2008. National health statistics reports. 2009; p. 1–14.
2. Mathias SD, Kuppermann M, Liberman RF, et al. Chronic pelvic pain: prevalence, health-related quality of life, and economic correlates. Obstet Gynecol 1996;87:321–7.
3. Reiter RC. A profile of women with chronic pelvic pain. Clin Obstet Gynecol 1990;33:130–6.
4. Abercrombie PD, Learman LA. Providing holistic care for women with chronic pelvic pain. J Obstet Gynecol Neonatal Nurs 2012;12:1–23.
5. Friedlander JI, Shorter B, Moldwin RM. Diet and its role in interstitial cystitis/bladder pain syndrome (IC/BPS) and comorbid conditions. BJU Int 2012;109:1584–91.
6. Marziali M, Venza M, Lazzaro S, et al. Gluten-free diet: a new strategy for management of painful endometriosis related symptoms? Minerva Chir 2012;67:499–504.
7. Santanam N, Kavtaradze N, Murphy A, et al. Antioxidant supplementation reduces endometriosis-related pelvic pain in humans. Transl Res 2013;161:189–95.
8. Barnes PM, Bloom B, Nahin RL. Complementary and alternative medicine use among adults and children. Hyattsville (MD): US Department of Health and Human Services, Centers for Disease Control and Prevention, National Center for Health Statistics, 2008. National health statistics reports. 2008; p. 1–23.
9. O'Hare PG 3rd, Hoffmann AR, Allen P, et al. Interstitial cystitis patients' use and rating of complementary and alternative medicine therapies. Int Urogynecol J 2013;24:977–82.
10. Bologna RA, Gomelsky A, Lukban JC, et al. The efficacy of calcium glycerophosphate in the prevention of food-related flares in interstitial cystitis. Urology 2001;57:119–20.
11. Theoharides TC, Kempuraj D, Vakali S, et al. Treatment of refractory interstitial cystitis/painful bladder syndrome with CystoProtek–an oral multi-agent natural supplement. Can J Urol 2008;15:4410–4.
12. Kallestrup EB, Jorgensen SS, Nordling J, et al. Treatment of interstitial cystitis with Cystistat: a hyaluronic acid product. Scand J Urol Nephrol 2005;39:143–7.
13. Figueiredo AB, Palma P, Riccetto C, et al. Clinical and urodynamic experience with intravesical hyaluronic acid in painful bladder syndrome associated with interstitial cystitis. Actas Urol Esp 2011;35:184–7 [in Spanish].
14. Van Agt S, Gobet F, Sibert L, et al. Treatment of interstitial cystitis by intravesical instillation of hyaluronic acid: a prospective study on 31 patients. Prog Urol 2011;21:218–25 [in French].
15. Shoskes DA, Nickel JC. Quercetin for chronic prostatitis/chronic pelvic pain syndrome. Urol Clin North Am 2011;38:279–84.
16. Katske F, Shoskes DA, Sender M, et al. Treatment of interstitial cystitis with a quercetin supplement. Tech Urol 2001;7:44–6.

17. Check JH, Cohen G, Cohen R, et al. Sympathomimetic amines effectively control pain for interstitial cystitis that had not responded to other therapies. Clin Exp Obstet Gynecol 2013;40:227–8.
18. Check JH, Cohen R. Chronic pelvic pain–traditional and novel therapies: part II medical therapy. Clin Exp Obstet Gynecol 2011;38:113–8.
19. Check JH, Wilson C, Cohen R. Sympathetic nervous system disorder of women that leads to pelvic pain and symptoms of interstitial cystitis may be the cause of severe backache and be very responsive to medical therapy rather than surgery despite the presence of herniated discs. Clin Exp Obstet Gynecol 2011;38:175–6.
20. Mazzola TJ, Poddar SK, Hill JC. Complex regional pain syndrome I in the upper extremity. Curr Sports Med Rep 2004;3:261–6.
21. Cai T, Luciani LG, Caola I, et al. Effects of pollen extract in association with vitamins (DEPROX 500®) for pain relief in patients affected by chronic prostatitis/chronic pelvic pain syndrome: results from a pilot study. Urologia 2013;80(Suppl 22):5–10.
22. Elist J. Effects of pollen extract preparation Prostat/Poltit on lower urinary tract symptoms in patients with chronic nonbacterial prostatitis/chronic pelvic pain syndrome: a randomized, double-blind, placebo-controlled study. Urology 2006;67:60–3.
23. Walczak JS, Price TJ, Cervero F. Cannabinoid CB1 receptors are expressed in the mouse urinary bladder and their activation modulates afferent bladder activity. Neuroscience 2009;159:1154–63.
24. Abrams DI, Couey P, Shade SB, et al. Cannabinoid-opioid interaction in chronic pain. Clin Pharmacol Ther 2011;90:844–51.
25. Lee SH, Lee BC. Use of acupuncture as a treatment method for chronic prostatitis/chronic pelvic pain syndromes. Curr Urol Rep 2011;12:288–96.
26. Zhu X, Hamilton KD, McNicol ED. Acupuncture for pain in endometriosis. Cochrane Database Syst Rev 2011;(9):CD007864.
27. Linde K, Witt CM, Streng A, et al. The impact of patient expectations on outcomes in four randomized controlled trials of acupuncture in patients with chronic pain. Pain 2007;128:264–71.
28. Elkins G, Jensen MP, Patterson DR. Hypnotherapy for the management of chronic pain. Int J Clin Exp Hypn 2007;55:275–87.
29. Anderson RU, Nagy TF, Orenberg E. Feasibility trial of medical hypnosis and cognitive therapy for men with refractory chronic prostatitis/chronic pelvic pain syndrome. UroToday Int J 2011;4:2–12.
30. van Ophoven A, Rossbach G, Oberpenning F, et al. Hyperbaric oxygen for the treatment of interstitial cystitis: long-term results of a prospective pilot study. Eur Urol 2004;46:108–13.
31. van Ophoven A, Rossbach G, Pajonk F, et al. Safety and efficacy of hyperbaric oxygen therapy for the treatment of interstitial cystitis: a randomized, sham controlled, double-blind trial. J Urol 2006;176:1442–6.
32. Tanaka T, Nitta Y, Morimoto K, et al. Hyperbaric oxygen therapy for painful bladder syndrome/interstitial cystitis resistant to conventional treatments: long-term results of a case series in Japan. BMC Urol 2011;11:11.
33. Zimmermann R, Cumpanas A, Miclea F, et al. Extracorporeal shock wave therapy for the treatment of chronic pelvic pain syndrome in males: a randomised, double-blind, placebo-controlled study. Eur Urol 2009;56:418–24.
34. Vahdatpour B, Alizadeh F, Moayednia A, et al. Efficacy of extracorporeal shock wave therapy for the treatment of chronic pelvic pain syndrome: a randomized, controlled trial. ISRN Urol 2013;2013:972601.

35. Wolsko PM, Eisenberg DM, Davis RB, et al. Use of mind-body medical therapies. J Gen Intern Med 2004;19:43–50.
36. Teixeira ME. Meditation as an intervention for chronic pain: an integrative review. Holist Nurs Pract 2008;22:225–34.
37. Grant JA, Rainville P. Pain sensitivity and analgesic effects of mindful states in Zen meditators: a cross-sectional study. Psychosom Med 2009;71:106–14.

Index

Note: Page numbers of article titles are in **boldface** type.

Obstet Gynecol Clin N Am 41 (2014) 511–520
http://dx.doi.org/10.1016/S0889-8545(14)00055-2 obgyn.theclinics.com
0889-8545/14/$ – see front matter

L

M

N

O

Q

S

T

U

V

Printed and bound by CPI Group (UK) Ltd, Croydon, CR0 4YY
03/10/2024
01040485-0014